Text Book on Dogs for Veterinary Graduates

Text Book on Dogs *for* Veterinary Graduates

Nityanand Pathak

B.Sc., B.V.Sc. & A.H., M.V.Sc., Ph.D., FNAVSI,
FANA, FMOBS, MAAVN
President, Pashu Chikitski Poshan Avam Kalyan Samiti
113B, Vatika, Sun City Vistaar, Izatnagar-243122, U.P.

SSPH

SATISH SERIAL PUBLISHING HOUSE
403, Express Tower, Commercial Complex
Azadpur, Delhi-110033 (India)
Phone : 011-27672852, Fax : 91-11-27672046
e-mail : info@satishserial.com, hkjain1975@yahoo.com
Website : www.satishserial.com

Published by :

SATISH SERIAL PUBLISHING HOUSE

403, Express Tower, Commercial Complex, Azadpur, Delhi-110033 (INDIA)
Phone : 011-27672852 Fax : 91-11-27672046
E-mail : info@satishserial.com, hkjain1975@yahoo.com

ISBN 978-93-86200-91-4

Cover Page suggested by Dr. S.K. Saha, PS, AN Division IVRI, Izzatnagar (U.P.)
Composed, Designed & Printed in India

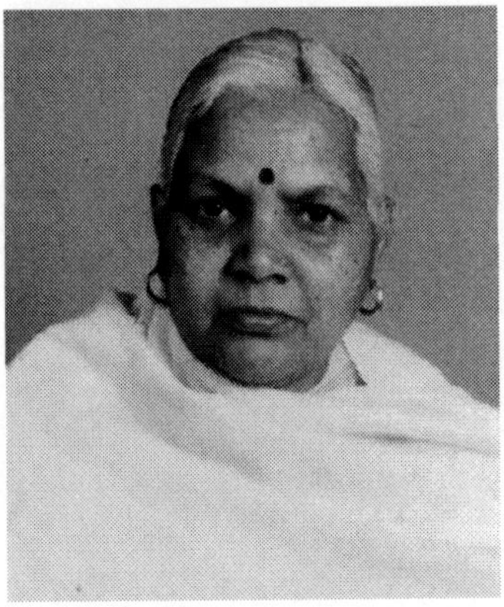

Dedicated to

Sushila

(18/06/1951 to 04/03/2004)

and

Her three pet dogs

Bulakee, Eam, and Gilloo

Preface

Dog (*Canis familiaris*) is a multipurpose domestic animal useful for all age group of humans without any bias for soical and cultural systems. It is an universal companion and different kinds of service providing animal from the beginning of the organized habitation of mankind. There are good books on the kinds of dogs but there appears to be no comprehensive book incorporating adequate informations on various aspects of dog as a subject of study of Veterinary courses. This book has been synthesized to meet the requirements of undergraduate/graduate veterinary students as well as guidance of dog owners and dog lovers. Dog keeping in India is different on many aspects, when compared with most of the Western countries.

By evolution dog is a carnivores animal which has been made omnivores after domestication and a step forward, it has been made milk based herbivores in the strict vegetarian Indian families. On incorporation uncommom foods from the pup life, the dogs develop taste for different kinds of area specific foods, fruits and vegetables. The book has been organized in 7 chapters comprising of the dog world, types of dogs, the morphology of dogs, reproductive system of dog and reproduction, digestive system of dogs, foods of dogs and nutrients supply and dietary management of sick dogs. The appendices include vaccination schedule, deworming schedule and glossary of the dog and kennel related terminologies. The list of terms used for dogs and kennel is one of the unique feature of this book, which are probably not in any book.

The book is educative also for the dog lovers, because few Indian dog owners try to learn details about the dogs. The number of nuclear families in continuously increasing and almost all eligible members are engaged for earning to run comfortable life. Under such circumstances, elders are left lonely in the house. In such situation requirement of companion dog is increasing. Therefore, it is also desired to aquire adequate informations about the behaviour and services of domestic dogs.

In the composition of this book, I was inspired by family members and pet dogs in the family. Thus, I take the opportunity to thank late Dileswari Devi and Ram Sakal Pandey (Buaji and Phuphaji), late Sushila and children. I also remember our pet dogs Moti, Kurzan, Bulaki, Eam and Gilloo for companionship. During processing of this book, I received help from Dr. Indrajit, L.C. Choudhary, V.B. Chaturvedi and Sri Harish

Chandra Singh in collection of photographs. My children Priyabhashini, Padmashini, Tripti and grand children Ananya, Anshuman, Anuvrata, Adya, Amuliya, Atharva, Anavartika and Akshita provided comfortable environment. Dr. S.K. Saha, Principal Scientist deserve special thanks for special interest in publication of this book.

Nityanand Pathak

About the Author

Prof. Nityanand Pathak, B.Sc., M.V.Sc., Ph.D., FNAVSI, FANA, FMOBS, MAAV has come from a small farming family of village Nagwa, district Ballia in Uttar Pradesh. He has served as researcher, teacher and extension personnel in India and ther country. At present he is President of Pashu Poshan Awam Pashu Kalyan Samittee and Indian Academy of Veterinary Nutrition and Animal Welfare, Bareilly. He has been President and General Secretary of Animal Nutrition Association, IVRI, Izzatnagar during 1995-1999 and foundation to 1995, respectively. He was President (2004-2006) and Vice President (2000-2002) of Indian Society of Animal Nutrition, NDRI, Karnal, Indian Society for Buffalo Development, CIRB, Hissar (2000-2002) and Indian Society of Zoo and Wieldlife Veterinarians, Bareilly and General Secretary of National Academy of Veterinary Science, India. He is recipient of first prize of Science Society, KKC-LU, 1961, Commonwealth Bureau of Animal Health Prize, 1969, New Surrey, England, Jawaharlal Nehru Award of ICAR, 1974, Institute level Best Teacher Award of IVRI, 1996, Meritorious Inovation Award, 2005 of the National Research Development Corporation, New Delhi and World Intellectual property Organization, Geneva-WIPO Award of Certificate of Merit, 2006. He is author and co-author of more than 350 research papers published in about 50 Indian and International Journals, many other scientific publications and 2 books and several other scientific publications. More than 150 scientific personnels has been co-authored and collaboration from the disciplines of Veterinary Medicine, Surgery, Reproduction, Livestock Management and Extension, etc.

About the Authors

Contents

Chapter 1

The Dog World

1.1 Introduction

Dog is perhaps one of the earliest companions of mankind that joined the development of civilization. In the process of the development of civilization, both needed each other which ultimately became a strong bond. The dogs participated in capture of food games and guarded developing inhabitation. During the progressive development of civilization, the dog became a loyal, agile, obedient and multi purpose pet. The modern domesticated dog is a highly refined animal and has been selectively breed to evolve in six broad groups for different purpose. In recent years, the demand of pet dogs, has increased greatly and it is expected to continue growing. Apparently most of the people think that keeping of a pet dog is very easy but it is not true, if someone really wants to keep the pet in standard/optimum management. Today, there are more than 500, breeds of dogs of six broad groups and ranging from less than 1 kg to almost 100 kg body weight. Therefore, it is essential for a novice family to make thorough assessment of self and family members before opting for keeping a pet dog in home.

1.2 Origin of Dog

For quite some time, the dog was considered to be evolved from wolves, jackal, coyate or foxes either independently through refinement by repeated selection or through cross breeding between these species in different combinations. The most accepted 3 theories are: (1) the ancestor of dog was wolf, (2) the dog was synthesized by cross breeding between wolf and jackal, or (3) the real ancestor of dog has now extinct. A fourth theory is that of a Charle's Darwin that states the dog was descended mainly from the two eastablished species of wolf. *i.e.* Canis lupus and Canis latrans and few other species of Indian, African and European origin, and South America besides few species of jackal and some similar extinct species. This needs further investigation for finding the true ancestors of modern dog.

1.3 Points to be considered before opting for dog keeping

It is very important specially for a novice desiring for keeping a pet dog. Some of the important aspects need critical analysis and consultation in the family. A decision to keeping pet dog(s) require consideration of physical, economic, social and psychological factors. In addition to these, one of the most important issue in some of the families is the willingness of acceptance by each one in the family.

1. First of all, it is important to ascertain the need of a pet dog in the home. It should be discussed at length among the adult family members living together in the same house. Children should also know about the plan of bringing a pet dog in the home. Following criteria may be considered during discussion among the family members regarding keeping a pet dog:
   - i) Acceptability of dog as a pet and level of acceptability.
   - ii) Behaviour of different family members with the pet. The pet dogs are very sensitive animal and desire affection and kindness.
   - iii) Extent of disliking, if any, by some of the members in family. Such problem is quite common in many Indian houses.
   - iv) Before taking decision for keeping a pet dog, assess that an old member or school going child is not burdened for unwilling managment of pet.
2. Very young and very old members in the family.
   - i) Most of the aged family members not exposed to a pet in home avoid handling because of unability or low acceptability.
   - ii) Infants and most of the children develop more affinity and proximity. This may be harmful for both, children and the pet.
3. To determine the purpose(s) of pet dog. This will help in selection of a suitable breed. Some of the common purpose of keeping a pet dog are :
   - i) A companion for the lonely person left alone in the house during duty hours.
   - ii) A companion-cum-guard for protection of household goods.

   iii) Herding the animals specially the flocks of sheep and goats.

   iv) Trailing and retrieving the games during hunting.

4. Assess the time sparable for the care and management of pet dog. This requires primary knowledge of different steps of dog management.

5. Self assessment for: (a) your expectations from the pet, (b) your ability to judge the actions of your pet for reward and punishment.

6. Food habits of family members and scope of flexibility in food habits or at least in the use of kitchen and few utensils for cooking the foods of pet.

7. Before selecting and procuring a pet dog, educate yourself and also take the family members in confidence for aquirying some basic knowledge about the general behaviour of the breed to be procured. Most of the toy breeds are agile, playful, affectionate and like the company of children, some of the medium sized like the company of sweet natured ladies and tall and large breeds like to remain at resting place during off hours.

8. Selection of an appropriate breed: It is very important to consider the selection of a breed according to covered and open space spared for the pet in the house. It will be inconvenient for the owner and the pet dog of large breeds to live in small apartments in thickly populated cities.

9. Body coat should be given special consideration due to the following reasons:

   i) Heat tolerence of double coat dogs is low and double coated breeds are less suitable. These breeds require adequate cooling arrangements during the hot summer months.

   ii) Double coated breeds need daily combing for keeping the coat free from mat formation and infestation of insects.

   iii) To collect loose undercoat for avoiding spread of fine fibres.

10. Hasty decision should be avoided in bringing the puppy for rearing as a pet.

11. After procurement per dog should be given necessary training for living in the house. These includes training for excretion

(urination and defecation), feeding at a predecided place and fixed time, obedience, barking against strangers but not snapping on the youngsters.

1.4 Points to be considered at the time of selection of puppy and later

The following points should be given due consideration at the time of selection of puppy and later:

1. The size and breed of the dog.
2. Purity of the breed: For the breeding programme pups should be selected from the pedigreed parent of the registered kennel club.
3. The puppy should be thoroughly examined for sex, teeth, physical appearance, toes, body coat and other factors.
4. The dog health card recording date of birth, parents, vaccinations and deworming, etc. must be obtained along with the puppy.
5. The pup should be procured at 5-6 weeks of age. It should be neither too young nor aged. Optimum age is 6 weeks, which is the end of nursing period.
6. Grooming should be scheduled at weekly interval in busy life but daily brushing/combing of coat and wiping of face, eyes, nose, ears and external genitalia is required.
7. Frequent bathing is not advised. The pet may be washed/bathed at monthly interval using an antiseptic soap or shampoo. However, dogs trained for birds hunting and fish catching should be given regular exposure for swimming in deep water and running in shallow water.
8. For pet dogs some essential training should be given from the early life. Use of rewarding and punishment is required for the proper training.
9. Training of defecation and urination outside the house should be strictly given. The dog should also not use the road, streets, parks and other public places.
10. The pet should be given a short name on the day of procurement and should be always called by its name.

11. The pup should be provided a rest box or basket at a fixed place in the house, if out, house or other place is not available. The place should be clean, dry, ventilated and cool, and it should not be exposed to hot sun and chilling wind. Exposure should be managed according to seasonal change in weather. Longer sun exposure may be given during winter otherwise exposure during exercise is adequate.
12. Sugars and sugar containing foods are normally not fed to dogs. Due to lack of sucrase dogs are unable to utilize sugars. But pet dog may develop sucrase producing ability. Probably sucrase secreting micro-organisms establish colonies in contact with human being.
13. All dogs require regular exercise. Large size and heavy breeds require rigorous exercise. Irregularity leads to indiscipline, besides introducing lethargyness, obesity and associated health problems.
14. Supplemental feeding should be introduced at 4-5 weeks of age. However, milk feeding may be necessary even from first or second week of age, if litter size is large.
15. Supplemental feeds are mostly based on milk and fed in the form of gruel and slurry in early life. Solid feeds are gradually introduced from 5-6 weeks of age.
16. Foods should be offered lukewarm.
17. Food should not be left for longer time for eating at will.
18. Time and place of feeding should be fixed.
19. Pet dog should not be allowed entry in kitchen.
20. It is highly undesirable to allow the pet to sit near the dining place and offer foods during dining.
21. Fruits, fruit juice, vegetables should be introduced in early life.
22. A good quality milk based baby food should be introduced at 5-6 weeks of age, if it is not possible to prepare slurry or puddings.
23. Feeding schedule of 4-5 meals daily at 5-6 weeks of age should be gradually reduced and fixed at 6 months of age for two (fore noon and after noon) times a day feeding at about 12 hours interval. Marginal adjustment of time may be made.
24. Meat is a natural food of dog. Cooked meat may be offered from 10-12 weeks of age. It is better to cook minced meat or spicules free fish with rice and leafy vegetables.

25. It is possible to maintain pets on milk based vegetarial foods provided care is taken for the balancing of nutrients. It is not advised to rear large and sporting breeds on meat free diets.
26. First deworming is normally done at about 6 weeks of age followed by a second dose after 3 weeks interval. Clinicians advise monthly deworming upto 6 to 12 months of age. Such practice should be ignored because use of drug is not good for health, as it causes stress on liver and kidneys for metabolism and elimination. Subsequent deworming should be done only in positive cases identified by faecal examination.
27. Vaccination must be done at right time advised by the veterinarian. Protection against rabies must not be delayed under any circumstances.
28. Male and female puppies should be separated before 6 months of age and should be provided separate pens or cubicles.
29. Puberty occurs at 9-12 months of age in different breeds, but breeding should be allowed at about 18 months of age.
30. Placenta is normally eaten by the bitch and it is a natural phenomenon.
31. Dogs do not need any clothing. It is inconvenient for most of the dogs and often harmful for the double coated breeds, reared in tropical countries.
32. Arrangements for examination and treatment of ailing dog should not be delayed to avoid complications and management problems.
33. If a pet is suffering from incurable disease, it is always humane to opt euthenetia. Unnecessary lingering is stressful for the dog as well as family members.
34. Dead pet should be disposed off honourably either by deep burial under the layer of lime or incineration.
35. Do not give calcium supplements during pregnancy and later to new born pups without consulting the veterinary doctor, otherwise structural deformities may occur in the litter.

1.5 Examination of Puppy / Dog before Procurement

It is always better to deal the procurement in free and frank environment because the dog is brought to live in the family almost life-long. Before procurement, the puppy or dog should be examined or got examined by a veterinary doctor for breed characters and soundness. The following guidelines may be followed for the physical examination of the dog before procurement:

1. General disposition: The animal should be observed for general condition and gait during walking. There should not be swing, staggering and lameness. The animal should stand in characteristic posture for the breed. The shape, size and body coat must meet the breed standard. The face should be carefully examined for scar at the level of cheek, teeth because extraction of tooth lives a scar mark. The face is also examined for loss of hairs and itching, etc.

2. Rectal temperature should be recorded of a resting animal. It should be 38-39 °C (100-102 °F) in most of the breeds and a little higher (40-42 °C or 104-108 °F) in hairless breeds.

3. Examination of oral cavity: The mouth is opened gently for examination and it is examined in light or help of torch may be taken. The palates, anterior part of pharynx, buccal surface of cheeks, dorsal surface of tongue, gums and teeth are examined fo the normal appearance. The nature of any abnormality like inflammatory changes should be got examined by a veterinarian for impact on the utility of dog. Preference should be given to healthy oral cavity without deficit of any tooth. The teeth in closed mouth should be characteristic (either level bite or scissor bite) for the breed. Only in few small face breeds, teeth may be undershot or overshot, and in other breeds these changes are deformity.

4. The eyes are examined carefully. These should be responsive, bright and attentive. Presence of opaque membrane on the pupil and any mark or scar on the cornea are not accepted. Dilated pupil is also a disqualification and it fails to contract on exposure to light. There should not be inversion of eyelids. This is observed by moist skin of lower eyelid. Special examination is required for the presence of a second row of eyelashes, which is frequently observed in Pekingese breed. It is a continued cause of irritation and such dogs should be avoided.

5. External ears or ear flaps should be characteristic for the breed and any change made by surgical intervention should be

informed before the examination. The ear flaps should not be puffy and inflamed. No fluid should flow out of the ear canal. The dog should also be examined for the normal hearing. This can be checked by response of the normal call of breeder from behind a wall or curtain. Good number of pure white dogs are born deef. It appears to be a hereditary disorder.

6. Nose colour should be characteristic for the breed. It should not be split down. The scar formed is rough and reduces the value of dog.
7. Examination of neck region: The fingers are moved carefully around the neck starting from the lower jaw to front of shoulders dorsally and upto brisket ventrally. The region should be smooth and free from any abnormal growth of lymph glands and abnormality (congenital or acquired) of cervical vertebrae.
8. Examination of thoracic region: The fingers are run along the thoracic region for the soundness of chest cage. There should not be bidding or exostoses.
9. Examination of abdomen and waist region: It is examined by moving the palms with gentle pressure on either side up to waist in normal standing position. The dog should not feel pain and abdomen should be soft. There should not be any palpable growth.
10. Examination of limbs: The dog is kept standing as far as possible in normal posture. The forelimbs are straight with close set and arched toes. Normally, there are one dew claw on the posterior aspect above the pastern. Sometimes, there may be more than one. The dew claws are generally cut off in early life without any problem. The hips are full and hind limbs are well- angulated. However, deflected forelimbs in Bull dogs and dropping hips in German Shepherd breeds are normal traits. There should not be erosion, cracks and corn like growth on the foot pads.
11. Examination of skin: It is examined by running the fingers through coat on the body for the detection of any abnormal growth, eruptions, crust formation, exudation and ectoparasitic infestations. Hairy and double coated dogs require careful examination.
12. Examination of coat: It should be characteristic for the breed, clean, glossy and free from greasiness. There should not be patches of alopacia and mat formation.

13. Examination of tail: The tail should be carried characteristic for the breed. As usual, it is examined by running the fingers close to vertebrae from base to tip. The common ailments are healed fractures and eviation from standard shape and size. The tail is lifted up for examining abnormalities of vent and gynecological ailment like prolapse, vulvo-vaginitis and tumour, etc. in the bitches.
14. In male dogs, scrotum is examined for the descending of testicles and prepuce is examined for phimosis and paraphimosis.
15. Examination of ventral aspect of body: The dog is secured properly and turned on its back at a smooth surface. The entire surface from brisket to groin is examined for scars, eruptions, abnormal growth and number of normal teats (in bitches only). Groin is checked for hernia.
16. Examination for locomotion and gait: The animal is led by a person and its gait and movements are observed for abnormalities.

There are no simple methods for the examination of internal organs. The external soundness of dogs is considered adequate for the procurement of a puppy/dog for rearing as a pet animal.

1.6 Signs of Health

It is important for the owners to have ampoule awareness for understanding the health status of their pet dogs. Some basic knowledge of common signs of health will be helpful in identifying the abnormal changes in appearance and behaviour of the dog. Thus, the pet dog should be examined daily for the following factors:

1. The dog should be active and alert, and should respond quickly to call.
2. Eyes, nostrils and body coat should display normal lusture.
3. Nose should be wet and glossy.
4. Gait should be normal and characteristic for the breed.
5. The response to food and water should be normal except that some times most of the animals escape a meal at interval of a week or two weeks, if it is not practiced by the owner.
6. Dullness and isolation at a secluded place require immediate attention, and may require clinical assistance. Quick veterinary

consultation will be always in the interest of the health of the dog and also for relief to owners from agony.

7. There should not be excessive (abnormal) salivation. Continuous drooling of saliva in string and non-responsiveness to owner's call may be suspected for the dangerous viral disease, rabies. Immediate steps should be taken for thorough clinico-pathological examination and further necessary action.
8. The tail should not be loose hanging except in the breeds of hanging tail.
9. Itching and foul smell from hairy breeds may be due to unnoticed skin ailments.
10. Bending and rubbing of ears should be suspected for otitis/ otorrhoea, if skin lesions are absent on the either surface and surrounding area of ear base.
11. Some cordinal signs of health may be observed by the owners themselves with a little training organized as part of social services by the veterinary doctors. There should be a clinical thermometer in each household and should be kept with grooming kit. Recording of pulse rate and respiration rate are specialized observations but owners should know the normal values.
12. Normal values of body (rectal) temperature, pulse rate and respiration rate of dogs are as follows:
    i) Body (rectal) temperature 38-39^{0}C. In some breeds, it is 41-42^{0}C.
    ii) Pulse rate (heart beat) per minute: The values are affected by age, sex and pregnancy (in pregnant bitches). The pulse rate is higher in pups and yearling and gradually decreases with the increase in age. The changes are relatively faster in large breeds.
        a) Values of pulse rate per minute

Pups and yearling	110-120	(115)
Adults	90-100	(95)
Aged (Geriatric)	70-90	(80)

        b) Values of normal respiration rate per minute

Pups and yearlings	18-20
Adults	15-18
Aged (Geriatic)	12-15

The ratio between respiration rate and pulse rate of health dogs is mostly 1:6. It is always better to register the pet in beginning with a veterinary clinic. This will be helpful in understanding the abnormalities in health from the history of the pet maintained at the clinic. Therefore, management of ailment may be easier and quicker.

1.7 Physical Properties of Dog's Faeces

Characteristics of fresh faeces are considered satisfactory indeces for the assessment of the health of digestive system and digestion of foods. The consistency of faeces has been used as a main factor for evaluation (Table 1).

Table 1. Grade of Physical Propertices of Faeces

Grade	Physical Properties of Faeces
1.0	Hard, solid, much dry, bullet like or spindle-shaped and non-sticky.
1.5	Hard, solid, less dry and non-sticky.
2.0	Normal well formed, kickable, does not leave soiling impression on removal from the floor. It may be a little sticky.
2.5	Well formed with slightly moist surface. It is slightly sticky and leaves soiling marks on the floor on removal. Immediate sweeping is needed.
3.0	Droppings are moist. Turns flat on falling and may further flattened, if removal is delayed for some time. It leaves definite soiling mark on the floor. Moderate sticky.
3.5	Loose but maintaining shape to greater extent. Complete removal from the floor require experience. Sweeping is needed.
4.0	Shape almost vanished, viscous due to loose consistency. Moderate stickyness. Removal requires skill. Early sweeping is essential.
4.5	Completely loose faeces without any shape and spreading on the floor. Its removal is difficult and requires sweeping into drain.
5.0	Completely watery and spreading (in case of severe diarrhoea). It is highly sticky and removed by sweeping only.

1.8 Assessment of Body Condition

The body condition of domesticated dogs can be assessed by visual examination in short body coat and by running the fingers close to body in long hair and double coat animals. Regular recording of body weight at an interval of 1, 2 or 3 months provides better information about the condition of dog provided, there is no change in behaviour and normal activities. Satisfactory assessment of body condition may be made by visual appraisal and palpation of the animal as shown in Table 2.

Table 2. Assessment of Body Condition of Domestic / Pet Dogs.

Body condition	Parameters to be observed
a) Thin/Sub-normal	1. Animal appears thin and weak.
	2. Ribs are visible in low coat dogs and can be felt by running fingers closed to chest and other parts of body in hairy and double coat dogs.
	3. Coccigeal vertebrae are visible in low coat dogs and can be felt depleted by running the fingers under the coat.
	4. Hip bones are visible in low coat dogs and as usual can be felt by running fingers in hairy/double coat dogs.
	5. Belly and waist are tucked up to various degree as per the degree of thinness. However, in most hounds it is a normal condition of body and should not be considered thinness or sub-normal condition.
b) Normal/Standard/ Ideal	1. Ribs can be felt only by putting light pressure.
	2. Coccigeal vertebrae are not visible and tail is smooth in appearance.
	3. Hip bones are not visible and smooth.
	4. Waist is almost smooth but belly is slightly tucked up on examination from sides.
	5. Neck is smooth and full.
c) Over weight/ Obese	1. Body appears dorsally round like barrel.
	2. Neck is heavily loaded and flabby due to thick layer of fatty tissue.
	3. Coccigeal vertebrae are enveloped in adipose layer.

4. Ribs are not felt due to layer of adipose tissue.
5. Belly and waist are almost fused and bulding.
6. Gait may be deviated from the normal and such dogs are reluctant to run and chase the games. Lying flat on sides or sitting idle is preferred.

1.9 Some notable Traits of Dogs

The dog is one of the early domesticated animal due to its liking and proximity with the mankind since the start of settling and civilization.

1. Domesticated as well as stray dogs prefer to live in the human habitations *viz.* villages, towns, lanes of human colonies, markets, streets of hotels and restaurants, railway station, bus stands and other places of human presence.
2. Pet dogs are good companion, guide, guard, chasing games, draught work assistance in search as a sniffer.
3. Sense of smell is about 40 times higher than the human. They are also capable of distinguishing familiar smell from the lots of mixed smells. This trait is highly developed in the sniffer breeds of dog. Services of sniffer dogs are used for the search and seizer of narcotics, explosives and intruders, etc.
4. Most of the breeds clearly differentiate black and white colour. However,many breeds have improved the sense of colour differentiation.
5. Dogs see more clearly in night than the human being.
6. Dogs are capable to cover almost 180° arc under their vision.
7. Auditory sense (hearing) of dogs is highly developed and they can hear and communicate from long distance.
8. Dog's family, pack or group quickly assemble for defence or aggression (if needed) on stress call from other member(s).
9. The command learning ability of most of the refined breeds ranges between 10 and 20 but some extraordinary intelligent dogs may grasp and follow upto 100 commands. These are highly valuable

super dogs. Such individuals are required to be put on regular practice. Similarly, there are some other individuals in the recognized efficient breeds which will never learn more than 5 commonds and few may be unruly to the extent that they will not care for the command in spite of awarding punishments. Such individuals are removed and disposed off.

10. The dogs are quite intelligent and capable to think like humans. Therefore, adequate and proper training are required for the better uses of dog's intelligence. Untrained dogs may be of little use for specialized works. Such dogs mostly remain as a show piece or create problem due to erratic behaviour in the absence of proper utilization.
11. Most of the dogs have extra sense of perception and capable of identifying the master of the family.
12. Pet dogs are normally hostile for the strangers and do not allow entrance in the premises, when free. Restrained dogs bark lowdly and attempt to snap.
13. Dogs communicate by barking, howling, whining and crying.
14. Pet dogs show affection by wagging tail, gazing at face, jollyfying movements and other playful actions.
15. Stray dogs have territorial behaviour and mark their territory by urination at different places along the boundary of its territory and do not allow the entry of other stray dogs.
16. Dogs are highly pain tolerant and whine when pain becomes intolerable.
17. Pet dogs generally do not like scolding and may be found to show displeasure by isolating away from the sight or avoiding eating. However, such reactions are short -lived and they respond quickly to gentle and affectionate call.
18. Sick dogs stop eating and try to hide in isolation at a dark place.
19. Free living yard dogs frequently dig the ground under shed for finding coolness during the hot summer season.
20. Anoestrous bitches do not permit mating and emit repelling odour.
21. Male dog showing aggression from a distance after sighting other stranger dog, turns polite and caring, when stranger dog is a bitch.

22. Pet dogs, living with human baby since its birth or early life, do not allow strangers to come near the baby even for showing love and affection to the baby.
23. Normally, dogs are not revengeful and selfish and do not fill guilty but exhibit fear or annoyance on scolding and punishing by beating. The bear the teeth and protest initially by begging vocalization and then by aggressive vocalization.
24. Some unruly dogs may snap on the children and ladies.

1.10 Sense of Smell in Dogs

This is one of the very important traits of dogs and due to this quality utility of sniffer dogs is increasing.

1. Newborn puppies are blind and deaf, and also unable to smell. The olfactory nerve and the smell centre of the brain are not fully developed. The sense of smell develops more rapidly than the sense of vision and hearing, as the later two are considered relatively less important than the sense of smell for the dogs.
2. The important activies and qualities of dogs are depends on the healthy and efficient nose.The sense of smell of dogs is highly developed. The odours of urine, sweat, blood, decomposing carcass, oestral discharge and anal glands secretion are basically interesting for the dogs.
3. The urine of a bitch contains a repellent substance which keeps male dogs away during the anoestrous period. The repelling substance is secreted by the luteal glands on the ovaries. On the onset of oestrous in bitches. The luteal glands synthesis of repellent. It is replaced by odours composed to stimulate and attract male dogs. It is commonly assumed that the male dogs can detect the oestral odours from a distance of several kilometers, but actually it is more likely that male dogs will be alerted by odour clues left by the bitch on her route or tracks while roaming. However, efficiency of male dogs can not be ignored as visiting of stray males near the housing of female in heat kept confined in house.

1.11 Expressions of Dog

For the development of good rapport with the dogs and faith of dogs in your attitude for them, it is important to understand the expressions of dogs. The dog is a pack animal and each member of a pack is assigned a position in hierarchy. This social system is strictly maintained by the members by changing posture in the presence of other members. The main signals are the facial expression, body posture and tail movements. Although there may be different kinds of expressions of minor differences but there are some distinct expressions to show reactions with the master and other family members, strangers and dogs of different groups.

The facial expressions of dogs may be differentiated into threat expression, fear expression, uncertain expression, affection expression, begging expression and subordiation expression.

1. **Threat expression:** This is an expression of warning to trespasser in the territory of dog. The trespasser may be a person, animal or some unusual newer article normally unknown to dogs. The threat may be firm, uncertain, mild, faint or casual. Younger dogs and nursing bitches are more reactive than the experienced dogs.

2. **Fear expression:** This expression is observed for the armed persons, horned cattle and buffaloes, kicking animals like horse, ass and mules, and the dominent dogs of other packs.

3. **Uncertain expression:** Such dogs are unpredictable and may be dangerous, as they can bite silently without warning or chasing.

4. **Affection expression:** It is always with the master and other family members. The pet looks eagerly and wags tail for appreciation and patting. They also want some playing and exhibit affection by the activities.

5. **Begging expression:** It is common in stray dogs of the locality and they visit door to door or in few houses for foods. They visit only those houses, where they get some food.

6. **Sub-ordination expression:** The dog bares teeth, pulls tail through groin to stuck with belly and bend down on hunches for pardon. The trapped outsider dog in a pack often lies down on back with folded drawn legs and ears in a posture of praying pardon for his mistakes. It may also happen within the pack for the correction of any unruly member.

1.12 Vocal Communication

The dogs communicate with other members of their pack and other packs by barking and howling in different narrations.

Whining and growling are observed among the littermates and also for communication with the mother.

Crying due to pain and weeping are also observed in the dogs. Weeping of dog is considered inauspicious and warning for some unwanted happenings.

1.13 Territory Marking

It is practiced by wild as well as domesticated canines. Urination at prominent projections along the habitation is a common practice. It is frequently renewed. A dog straying away from the pack or locality due to some reasons go on urinating at short intervals. This marking is used for returning to pack/home.

1.14 Behaviour of Dogs

The domestic dogs are generally kept as a pet animal for performing variety of activities. In India, the number of pet dogs in the boundry of homes is much less than the number of tamed stray dogs distributed from the lanes and streets of human habitation colonies to markets, restaurants, bus stands, railway stations and other public place with scope of availability of food refuses. Stray dogs live in groups and limit their movements in their own territory except during the breeding season. Since population of stray dogs is spread in almost all human inhabited areas in India, it is very important to have basic knowledge about the behaviour of stray dogs and the dogs in confinement.

1.15 Importance of Dog Behaviour

Although dog is considered to be domesticated first and also, a royal companion of mankind, but sray dogs are mostly unpredicted. Most of the stray dogs do not like strangers (man or animals) in their territory. The entrance of outsider provokes the first dog in sight and the specific call takes no time to collect the others and chase away the intruder(s) or to continue protest, if intruder is stroger. Incidence of attack and biting by stray dogs specially during dark hours of night is very common. The children and ladies are easy victims. Some of the general behaviour of domesticated (pet and street) dogs are listed as follows:

1. The dog is a social animal and even street dogs prefer to live in the human habitations and also with domestic animals. Probably food security, safety and congenial very long association are the factors governing such behaviour.
2. All dogs are very sensitive and pet dog knows every person, animals and articles in the house and also the persons frequently visiting the house. The dog on arrival of such persons at the door-step simply acknowledge that he is aware of Even the street dogs know the behaviour and foot-steps of residents of their locality and do not show any reaction or moves tail affectionately or follows upto door-step of the resident. Most of the dogs also accept the accompanied stranger(s). Methods of vocalization are different for the residents and strangers.
3. Street dogs also develop unbound relationship with all the residents of their territory and do not show any aggressive reaction in daytime and even in the dark hours, gives a mild warning from a distance but immediately becomes calm after recognizing the foot-steps and finally the person. Some street dogs often follow-upto doorstep of the resident.
4. The street dogs react sharply with the strangers and start roaring,barking and giving call to others for chasing or challenging the stranger. This reaction alerts the residents for finding the reasons for their vocalization. Street dogs are unpaid guards of the colony providing services on kitchen residues only.
5. Perhaps dogs are unable to see clearly or recognize a person from long distance beyond 7 metres. These dogs also recognize the sound of vehicles to greater accuracy.
6. There is also some opinion that the dogs are weak in differentiating colour but I am fully convinced that the dogs are capable of identifying many colours.
7. The olfactory organs of dogs are highly developed and they are capable of not only smelling a substance from very long distance but they are also capable of differentiating the different smells. The sense of smell of a dog is considered to be about 100 times more than the smelling power of mankind human.

1.16 Measures of Behaviour in Dogs

Domesticated dogs are found friendly with the known humans and animals. Out of different types of wild dogs, only those frequenting the human habitations could be domesticated. Such dogs continue to live in human proximity even after abondonning stray. However, for effective utilization of dogs; services, general training is given for observing normal descipline and works. Special rigorous training is given to the selected highly intelligent members of the lots for highly technical jobs. Therefore, it is important to have adequate knowledge about the behaviour of dogs. The important parameters used for the measurement of behaviour of a domestic dog including the stray dogs of human habitation are as follows:

1. Aggression
2. Affection
3. Expulsion
4. Playful
5. Unmindful or indifferent
6. Barking

Table 3. Some Breeds more liked by ladies

Breed	Countries
Bichon	France
French Bulldog	France
Lowchen	France
Poodles	France, England
Italian Greyhound	Cleoptra owned one. Patrician ladies.
Japanese Chin	Japan (Often carried in the sleeves of kimonoa)
Lhasa Apso	Many countries
Maltese	Greek and Roman ladies

1.17 Average Longivity of Domesticated Dogs

Various factors are responsible for the longivity of domesticated dogs. Climatic conditions and management are the main factors affecting the longivity of domesticated dogs. Observations and experience say that an increase in the shape and size reduces the longivity. Some tentative values of longivity of dogs of different size groups are given in Table 4.

Table 4. Tentative values of longivity of domesticated dogs of different size.

Body size class	Body weight (kg)	Longivity (Years)	Average life (years)
Heavy breeds	More than 35	8-12	10
Upper medium breeds	20-35	10-15	12
Medium breeds	10-20	12-18	14
Small breeds	5-10	15-20	17
Toy or tiny breeds	Less than 5	15-25	20

1.18 Dogs in Mythology

India: The ride of Hindu God Bhairav is a black dog. "Bhairav" is a devotee of Goddess "Durga".

At the end of Mahabharat war King Yudhisthir refused the offer of heaven without his pet dog and subsequently, the dog was also allowed.

Celestial dog (Tien-Kou): The dog which helped the second Lord (Erh-lang) in driving away the evil spirits (page 382 of New Larousse Encyclopedia of Mythology, Prometheus Press, Paris).

In Uganda, "the bad treatment of a dog made situation for awarding death to man.

1.19 Some Important Dates and Events in the History of Domestic Dogs

1. Saluki is the first defined breed of domestic dogs by the Arabs.
2. Some basic behaviours remaining unchanged by domestication and selection:
   i) Wagging of tail as an expression of behaviour.
   ii) Territory marking by male dogs with urination at prominent places.
   iii) Growling on strangers (human, animals including dogs).
3. Dogs were primarily domesticated for hunting, guarding and companionship.

4. First Dog Show was held in 1859 at Newcastle Upon Tyne in England. The show was only for the hunting dogs and 50 enteries were encouraging.
5. English Kennel Club was established in 1873.
6. American Kennel Club was established in 1884.
7. Italian Kennel Club was established in 1898.
8. International Leonberger Club was started in 1895 at Stuttgart, Germany.
9. Klub der deutschen Boxer-Freunde (Boxer Friends Club) was established in 1896 in Germany.
10. Verein fur deutsche Schaferhunde (German Shepherd Dog Society) was started on 22nd April, 1899 at Stuttgart, Germany.
11. Federation of Cynologique International (FCI) was founded in 1911.
12. First informative book on dogs was written by Xenophon during 430-352 B.C.
13. At present, dog breeds are more than 500 and many breeders are still engaged in evolving synthetic breeds of desired traits by incorporating germplasm of several breeds.
14. In India, some high dog breeds are helpful/careful for Police, Army, CISF, CRPF and other security forces for the security of national *i.e.* against terrorism, security of bus-stands, railway-stations, metro-stations, borders and also dogs are helpful for find criminals and suspicious articles.

❑❑❑

Chapter 2

Types of Dogs

The dogs are though the earliest domesticated animal considered to be domesticated during the stone age but still different types of wild dogs are found in the forests and hilly regions. There are also dogs that escaped with wild dogs and became feral. Classification of dogs can be done by different ways.

2.1 Classification of Dogs on the Basis of Habitat

Dogs can be divided into four groups on the basis of habitat. These are wild dogs, feral dogs, domesticated dogs and mongrels or street dogs.

i) The Wild Dogs

The wild dogs are often referred as feral dogs, which is not a correct identification. Almost all kinds of remaining wild dogs prefer to live away from the human habitations They are mostly pack animals and maintain a social organization based on hierarchy. The different kinds of wild dogs are found in the Africa, Asia-Europe region, America and Australia. All wild dogs are not included in the genus Canis.

ii) The African Wild Dogs

As expected, it is a carnivorous wild animal found mostly in deciduous thin forests and savannah inhabitating different species of wild ungulates, rodents and other animals for the assured supply of carcass for food. The dogs live in pack and mostly hunt small and medium size antelope, deer and other animals. Now, it is an endangered species included in IUCN.3.1 of 2008.

Zoological classification of African Wild Dog (Fig. 2.1)

Kingdom	Animalia
Phylum	Chordata
Class	Mammalia

Order	Carnivora
Family	Canidae
Sub-family	Caninae
Genus	Lycaon
Species	Lycaon pictus
Sub-species	L.P. Pictus
	L.P. Lupinus
	L.P. Manguensis
	L.P. Somalicus

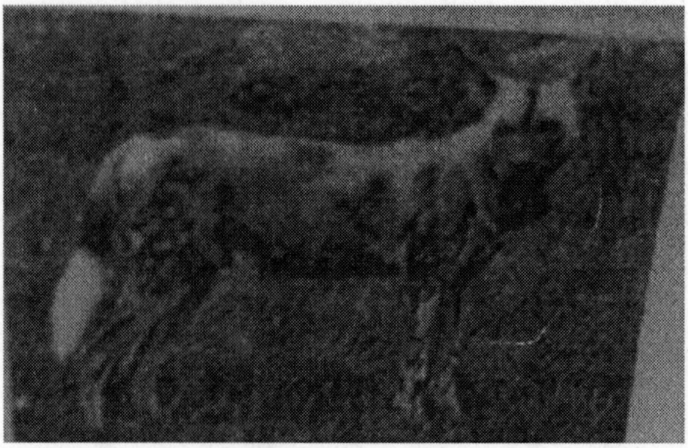

Fig. 2.1 African wild dog

The zoological name Lycaon pictus has been synthesized from a Greek word "Lycaon" means wolf and a Latin word "pictus" for the painted subject. In some of the literatures, the name Canis pictus has been also used.

Synonyms of African Wild Dogs

There are many synonyms of the African Wild Dog. The English names are: 1. The African Hunting Dog, 2. The Cape Hunting Dog, 3. The Painted Hunting Dog, 4. The Painted Wolf and 5. The Spotted Dog. In African language, it is called Wildehond and in the Swahili language, it is Mbwamwitu. The name African Wild Dog is repulsive for many groups and it has been suggested to use Painted Hunting Dog. However, the name African Wild Dog has been used in this chapter for the Lycaon pictus and not to hurt the feelings of anybody.

Morphology of the African Wild Dog (Lycaon pictus)

The African wild dog is medium to large size animal with some regional variation. The dogs in south part of Africa are larger than the dogs in other parts. This genus has been differentiated from the other canids due to absence of dewclaws on the forelegs. Although clear sexual dimorphism is generally ignored but in captivity, the males have been found a little larger than the females of same pack. The dog is tall measuring about 75 cm. at the shoulder. The body length from head to base of the tail is about 100 cm. and the long bushy tail ranges from 30 to 45 cm. Body weight of adult dogs is most variable and ranges from 17 to 36 kg.

Adult dogs contain 42 teeth comprising of 6, 2, 8 and 4 number of incisors, canines, premolar and molar teeth, respectively on the upper jaw, and 6, 2, 8 and 6 for the corresponding type of teeth on the lower jaw, as depicted in the following dental formula:

Dental formula of permanent teeth = I 3/3 C 1/1 P 4/4 M 2/3 = 10/11 X 2 = 42.

The premolar teeth are larger than the other canids and suitable for consuming more bones. The other important feature enabling higher shearing capacity and faster eating of prey is the single cusp crested first lower molar tooth. The condition is called trenchant heel. The bite force quotient (BFQ) means the strength of bite measured against the body mass of an animal, is 142 and it is highest amongst the different carnivora species. The BFQ is a measure for the assessment of predatory traits of the carnivorous animals.

Social Organization Pattern in African Wild Dogs

The African wild dogs live in packs and the size of packs depends on the number of females, their followers and male mates. Within the packs, the hierarchy is different for the bitch and the male. The position of head of the group is called the alpha position and it is occupied by the senior most bitch over other bitches including the daughters. In case of death of the alpha bitch, the successor will be the next senior most bitch in the pack. Split in the pack is common and separate groups are formed by the bitches of equal status after the death of alpha bitch. The system of occupying alpha position in the male dogs is different and an younger male in the family or from the other family may form a joint larger pack.

The African wild dogs are not aggressive by nature with in the community and hierarchy system in the pack is submission based and not the dominance based. Fighting is not acceptable and the packs are managed by amicable behaviour of submission and non-aggression. One of the main factor for the evolution of submission based hierarchy is the food and protection requirements for the rearing of large size litter of upto 19 puppies in some superior mothers. Sometimes, an unrelated male joins a pack for short time and in very rare case, an unrelated male attempts to occupy alpha position by aggression.

During the outing of packs for hunting the mother and pups and also the sick, injured and aged members are left behind in the den. The hunting in packs results almost 80 per-cent successful in killing the prey. In the cursorial system of hunting, the packs chase the prey long on the open grasslands. The chasing of prey is co-ordinated by characteristic vocalization to communicate with each other in the pack. The sound made during chasing the prey is different. It is chirping or squeaking like the terrestrial birds for alarming the members in the flock.

The killed object is eaten by the pack and most of members eat more for carrying back to den. On return from hunting, some of the injested meat is regurgitated for feeding the members left behind in the den. Although some difference may be observed in the selection of prey by different packs but majority find medium size ungulates more easy. Sometimes, large size running birds are also hunted. The killed object of dog packs is some times stolen by the other predators like lions.

The large packs of African wild dogs some times venture for hunting large beasts like zebras. This requires close co-ordination skill. The pack members first observe the movement of herd and move nearer the herd while hiding themselves in the tall grasses. After signal of the alpha or co-ordinator, the suddenly charge to create panic resulting in stamped in the herd. At this stage, one of the animal is caught by tail and immediately another dog catches the upper lip. Simultaneously, other members of the pack attack the prey and it is downed on the ground. This approach is also used for the killing of wild buffaloes, large size antelope and young girrafe. It is believed that African wild dogs start eating the prey even it is live. Due to this behaviour, Lycaon pictus was considered repulsive. However, some recent observations claim that prey of African wild dog die more quickly than the prey hunted by big wild cats like the lion and the leopard. The method of hunting large ungulates appears to be art, developed by some of the packs and followers of the pack are given perfect training for hunting.

Reproduction in African Wild Dogs

Both sexes of the African Wild Dogs attain maturity for fertile breeding at 12 to 18 months of age. There is no seasonality of breeding and it occurs round the year. But rate of breeding is more during the later half of the rainy seasons in the month of March and June. The corresponding period of whelping is May and August. Gestation period is about 70 days. Average litter size has been found 10 but variation is very wide and ranges from 2 to 19 pups in a litter. The pregnant bitch search some abandoned den by other animals in the vicinity of her habitat for whelping. Care is taken to select well, protected place for whelping. The nursing bitch live behind the pups under the care of other members of the pack. Weaning occurs at about 10 weeks of age. During this long nursing period, the bitch and her pups are fed vomitus of other members of pack. Next mating normally takes place at an interval of 12 to 14 months but it can be shorten to about 6 months in case of early death of litter, still births and abortions. After about 3 months of whelping, the den is deserted by the family and the pups are put on training to gradually move with the pack and learn the art of chasing and hunting the prey. The pups start hunting small prey at 8-10 months of age and become capable of organizing hunting with packmates.

The female pups after attaining maturity generally leave the mother's pack at 15 to 30 months of age to join the group of eligible bachelors for forming their separate pack. Males rarely abandon the original pack. It means the new packs are generally formed by the mature bitch perhaps for establishing her hierarki. The bitch select a mate that will take care of pups in early life and bring food for the family. In a normal pack, males are almost double in number. This dog is very much conscious about the growth and only dominant bitch breeds in a pack.

Distribution of African Wild Dog

Natural distribution of the animals is limited in the Africa and these are present all over the countries, where wild animals particularly the ungulates are found. Some of the factors determining the presence are the size of packs, availability of prey, absence or rare presence of other predators and availability of safe dens. Once distributed in about 39 countries of Africa, now it has been shrunken to only 14 countries or so.

The countries providing protection for conservation and research are the Tanzania (Selous Game Reserve), Botswana, Namibia, South Africa (Kruger National Park), Kenya, Mozambique and Zimbabwe, etc.

iii) The Indian (Asian) Wild Dog or Dhole (Cuon alpinus)

It is a red colour dog almost similar to the domesticated dog. They are ferocious but not scared of human. Like other canids, Dhole also live in packs developed of the family. These are highly efficient predator and even the big wild cats (lion, tiger, panther and leopard) normally avoid the Dhole packs.

Synonyms of the Indian Wild Dog

The wild dog has been given several regional names like Asiatic Wild Dog, Red Wild Dog, Red Indian dog, Kuong-kukur (North-East states of India), Ranga-kukur (Assam), Earam-naiku (Gujarati),Ban-kukur or Ban kuta (Bengal), Jungali-kutta, Ramhun, Ban kutta, Bhansa (Kashmiri), Kattu Naya, Chennaya (Malyalam), Chen Nai (Telugu), Kado Nayi (Kannada),Vana Kooka (Telugu), Adivi-kutta, Sone-kutta, Sona kukur (Hindi) and Ban Kukur (Gorkhali).

Zoological classification of Indian wild dog (Fig. 2.2)

The place of Indian wild dog in animal kingdom has been identified as follows:

Kingdom	Animalia
Phylum	Chordata
Sub-phylum	Vertebrata
Class	Mammalia
Sub-class	Eutheria
Order	Ungulata
Sub-order	Carnivora
Family	Canidae
Genus	Canis
Species	Familiaris (Canis familiaris)

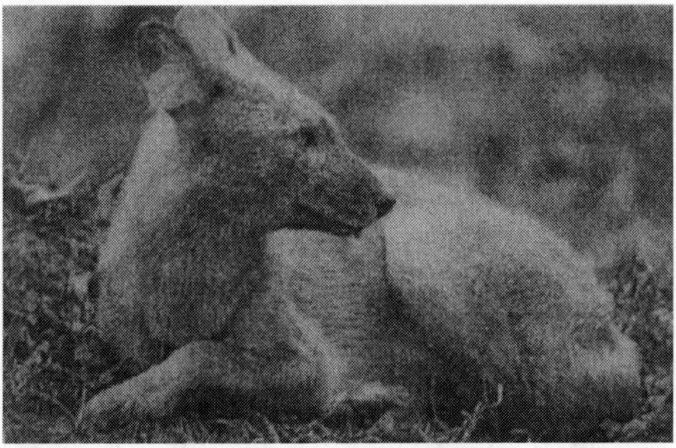

Fig. 2.2 Indian wild dog

Morphology of the Indian/Asian Wild Dog/Dhole

It is a medium, sized dog similar to most of the native stray dogs of the region. The body coat is reddish and hair length is variable in different regions.The tail is bushy and black. There is visible sexual dimorphism in the packs. The males are taller and larger than the females. The long face is formed of almost equal length of frontal and nasal bones with distinct stop. The ears are slightly tilted outwards near the somewhat rounded tip. Body weight ranges from 10 to 13 kg for the adult bitches and 15 to 20 kg in the adult males. Average body length from head to root of the tail is about 90 cm. and height at the shoulder is about 60 cm.

Structure of the Packs and Reproduction

The Indian Dhole lives in packs in the deep forest and hilly forest upto 2100 m height. The selection of habitat generally depends on the availability of food animals, water sources, open grass cover with woodland and serub for hiding. There should not be burrows of enemies like hyana and porcupine, dens of lion, tiger and other big cats and human interference due to their habitation.The packs are mostly the family of single pair containing 5 to 12 members of different age. Larger packs of upto 25 members of two or more families are also seen. The nursing bitches live with the offsprings for guarding and two to three dogs bring foods for the nursing bitch and her pups. The food is as usual offered by regurgitation.

Reproduction is highly controlled and only dominant male and dominant bitch at alpha position reproduce. This behaviour appears to has been evolved for the better care of replacement progeny to produce efficient predators. Whelping takes place in a den or burrow at a protected place. It is not uncommon to put another adult member of pack for guarding the pups in burrow, when mother sometimes join the hunting pack.

Sexual maturity is normally attained at about 12 month of age. Breeding is mostly seasonal from September to February. Gestation period (60-62 days) in Dhole is similar to domestic dogs. The pups are weaned at about 8 weeks of age but continue to live with the mother and trained for developing hunting skill during outing with the pack. Most of the dogs die before 10 years of age but may survive upto 16 years in captive housing in the zoos.

Distribution and Present Status

The Dhole dogs are found in deep forests with grasslands carrying different species of ungulates and other food animals for prey in the Indian sub-continent, Myanmar, Thailand, Combodia, Vietnam, China, Korea, East part of Russia and the island countries of Asia-Pacific region like Indonesia and Malyasia, etc.

The Dhole is almost extinct from the north-east hill states of India excluding the Assam due to extensive hunting for table purpose. These are occasionally reported in the forests of northern districts of West Bengal and adjoining forests and frequently seen in remote areas of Arunachal Pradesh and Garo hills of Meghalaya. The situation is not much different in Vietnam and many parts of China. There may be small packs in the sub-Himalayan forests. In southern states of India, Dhole packs have been sighted in the forests and hilly regions of the Kerala, Karnataka, Andhra Pradesh, Maharashtra, Madhya Pradesh and other states. There appears to be no recent statistic of Dhole packs. However, some packs are protected in different wildlife reserves in India and Nepal.

Three types of wild dogs are claimed to be present in Australia. These are dingo, feral domestic dogs and hybrids of the two. Among the three types, dingo may be considered as true wild dog of Australia which is claimed to be introduced from Asia about 4000 years ago. Wild dogs are menace for livestock due to predation of large number of farm animals on grazing lands.

iv) Australian Wild Dog or Dingo (Fig. 2.3)

Dingo is a medium-sized dog measuring 48-58.5 cm. (19-23 inches) at shoulders and weighing 23-32 kg (50-70 pounds). Exceptionally, large dingoes upto 55 kg (120 lb) has been reported. Yellow-ginger colour coat is soft and dense. The colour, length and texture of body coat change with the climatic changes in different season. Other less common coat colour are dull brown, tan, black and white. Rarely albino and brindle may be seen. Well feathered long tail is bushy and carried semi-coiled at higher level than the back. The face is moderate and medium size mobile pricked ears are rounded at the tip. The neck is short. Hind quarters are strong, lean and muscular. Dewclaws are absent in dingo. The head is mostly in line with the dorsal line. Face is demarketed by clear stop at the level of inner canthus. The eyes are sharp and yellow to orange in colour.

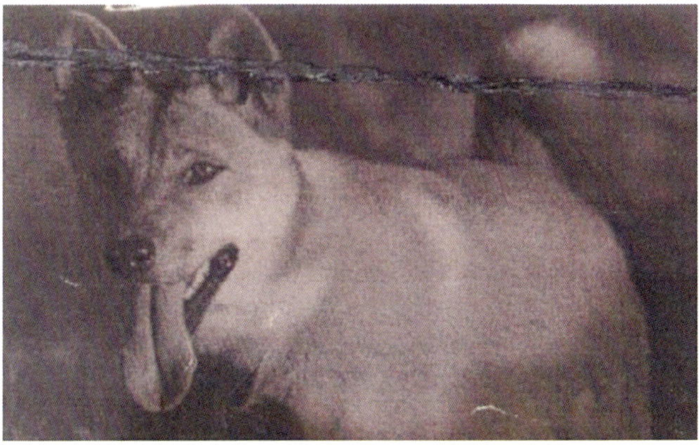

Fig. 2.3 Australian wild dog or dingo

The dingo can climb on different types of trees and sometimes likes isolated living. The dingo bitches breed only once annually and choosing of life-long partnership is characteristic. They mourn the death of partner. The hollow of large tree or similar place is used for whelping. The site is protected from three sides and front is watched by the dam.

v) The Pariah Dog (Fig. 2.4)

The word "Pariah" is used for the lower category of families in Tamil language and it has been used for describing the feral dogs of comparable phenotype distributed in India and many countries of Asia-Pacific region. It is not a well-defined type and several varieties are still found. All Pariah dogs are feral and live near the human habitation, but all feral dogs are not Pariah.

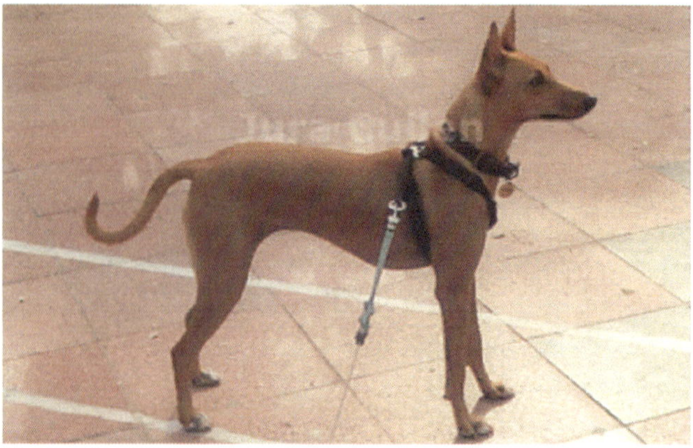

Fig. 2.4 Pariah dog

Synonyms of Pariah Dog

Pi dog, pye dog, feral Indian dog, Asiatic feral dog, primitive dog, etc. There is great variation in the morphology of pariahs of different countries and different regions. Unlike dhole, the pariah dogs are found near the human habitations and due to this reason, purity has been disturbed in the countries like India, where large number of street dogs are widely distributed.

Morphology of Pariah Dog

The pariahs are medium-sized dog with pricked ears, sharp eyes, moderately feathered tail, broad chest and moderately tucked up abdomen. Purebred utility pariah dog has been registered in USA kennel. It has been found very efficient for chasing large games. Many sports and utility breeds have been developed in different countries from the local strains of pariah dogs.

vi) The Carolina Dog/ American Dingo (Fig. 2.5)

It has been found from the paintings and rock depiction of ancient dogs by native American is morphologically similar to wild Carolina dogs living away in woodland and near swamps away from the human habitation.

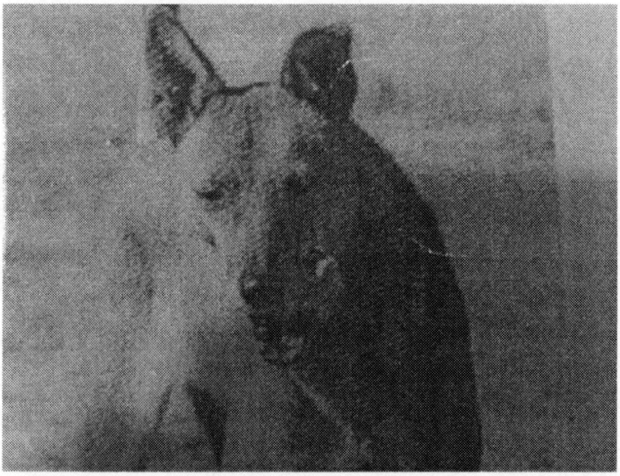

Fig. 2.5 Carolina Dog / American Dingo

Synonyms

Dixie Dingo, Indian Dog, North American Native Dog, Yaller Dog and Yellow Dog.

Description

This wild dog was not known due to its habitation in woodlands and grasses near swampland in southern region of United States of America far away from the human habitations. These are medium-sized dogs of 45-61 cm (17-24 inches) height and 15-20 kg (30-44 lb) body weight. Body coat is mostly fawm of different intensity. Dark colour mask is quite common. The dog resembles dingoes.

In Carolina bitches, three successive oestrus cycles occur in the breeding season. Probably, it was a natural arrangement for whelping during the healthy season for providing protection to neonate puppies before the emergence of diseases. Loss of puppies due to heart worm is often heavy. Many pregnant bitches have been found to dig dens for protected whelping. They also dig through soil for covering excrements. Digging of snout pits of muzzle size in soil is quite common and bitches dig more holes than the dogs.

Hunting behaviour of Carolina dogs is highly co-ordinated and specific pack formation during chasing the prey is highly effective for capturing. During chasing the trail, the motion is whip like swirling.

Carolina Dogs can be registered with American Rare Breed Association (ARBA) as a primitive dog.

Wild Dog of South America or Peruvian Wild Dog or Bush Dog of Peru.

This dog is distributed over a large area in the central zone of South America covering several countries. Little is known about the behaviour and characteristics of the wild dog of Peru, because it lives in forests and savannah. It is a medium-sized carnivorous dog thrives on capturing large rodents. Sometimes, they also eat small amount of fruits and leaves. Bush dogs mostly live in the group of family members.

vii) The New Guinea Singing Dog (NGSD)

This wild dog of New Guinea island has been found to be present since the stone age. The dog is described as a living fossil moving on four foots in the New Guinea island. The territory of this wild dog remained confined for thousands of years in the boundary of New Guinea island. The NGSD live in upland and thrive on hunting. First time, it was moved out of New Guinea island during 1954 to Australia but they escaped. Subsequently, another group was translocated in 1956 and used for multiplication. The dog is highly intelligent but does not like captivity. Only with rigorous training and close habitation in the vicinity of human habitation.

Characteristic Vocalization

Unlike common dog (Canis familiaris) the NGSD are able to howl like a wolf but distinctly different from wolf, the NGSD modulates the pitch of voice in a melody form. Due to this unique quality of vocalization, this dog has been given the name Singer or New Guinea Singing Dog.

Other Names

New Guinea Singing Dog (NGSD), New Guinea Highland Dog, Singer Dog.

Zoological classification of NGSD (Fig. 2.6)

Kingdom	Animalia
Phylum	Chordata
Class	Mammalia
Order	Carnivora
Family	Canidae

Genus	Canis
Species	Lupus (Canis lupus)
Sub-species	C l hallstromi

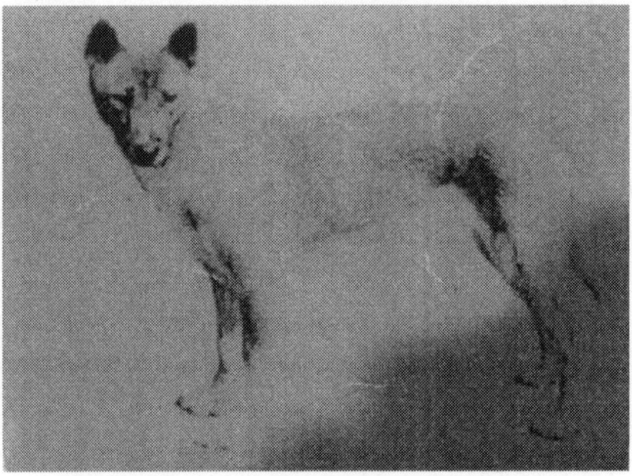

Fig. 2.6 New Guinea Singing Dog

Description

Perhaps no information is documented about the general characteristics, behaviour. The NGSD appears like a fox to greater extent. The dog is covered with double coat of red to brown colour. Some dogs may have melanistic mask. The upper first molar or characteristic carnassial tooth is extraordinary large. Height at shoulders ranges from 36 to 46 cm (14 to 18 inches) and body weight range is 8 to 14 kg (17 to 30 lb). The head is relatively larger and legs are shorter than the other wild dogs. Pricked front facing ears are placed apart on the relatively wider skull. The dog possesses high drive for hunting. Although gentle and affectionate but does not like confinement and control. Digging and climbing are attempted for escaping.

Some other relatives of dogs or canids grouped with the dogs are: (i) the Bush Dogs (Speothos venaticus) of South America, (ii) the Raccoon Dog (Nyctereutes procyonoides) of Asia and (iii) the Small Eared Dog (Atelocynus microtis) of South America.

viii) Domesticated Dog (Canis familiaris)

Domesticated dogs have been evolved for variety of performances in the advanced countries of Europe, America, Japan, Australia and some other small countries. Synthesis of breeds was related with the prosperity of the nations. The domestic dogs of such countries are maintained in controlled housing. However, in economically developing countries, domesticated dogs live in different conditions. The domesticated dogs living in the conditions of Indian sub-continent may be distinguished in the following classes:

1. **Kennel dogs:** These are well-defined pedigreed animals registered with the Kennel Club of the country. These are exclusively kept for commercial breeding, participation in dog show and other exhibitions.
2. **Tamed dogs:** These are street dogs breeding in a locality. These dogs are not housed but fed by the families living in the colony. Almost all family members are the owner of these dogs.
3. **Yard dogs:** These are also undefined breeds of local dogs born in the yard and consider the yard their home. Although these dogs are not restrained and roam freely but invariably arrive at the time of meals and rest in the courtyard. These are good guards for livestock and households.
4. **Field dogs:** These are also free living but patronized dogs. These are fed by the farmers. In morning, the dogs take morning meal and then accompany the farmer to field and stay with owner the whole day. On the farms, these dogs protect crops from stray cattle. These dogs return back with owner.
5. **Field crop guard dogs:** These are also patronized dogs that are maintained by vegetable growers and orchard owners for the protection of crops from stray and wild animals and also prevent theft.
6. **House dogs:** These are mostly pedigreed dogs either purchased from a registered kennel club or received gift from a friend or relative. These may or may not be a trained dog. These are mostly guard and companion dogs. Some of the popular breeds are German Shepherd, Labradoe, Dobermann Pinscher, Pomeranian, Samoyed, Gaddi, Bhotia and Dalmatian.

2.2 Classification of Dogs on the Basis of Geographical Distribution

1. **Dogs of arctic and sub-arctic zones :** These are generally upper-medium-sized dogs of strong built with bonned limbs suitable

for hunting food animals and pulling sledge. The body is covered with doble coat. The under coat is dense, soft and short. The outer coat is long and dense and does not allow percolation of water to wet under coat.

2. **Dogs of temperate zone :** There is great variation in the dogs of temperate and sub-temperate region. Perhaps largest number of breeds have been synthesized in the Europe and United States of America. These are mostly double coated dogs ranging from less than 1 kg to more than 70 kg body weight.
3. **Dogs of tropical zone:** The dogs in free living form are mostly short-haired and medium-sized animals with scanty coat on the ventral aspect of body extending from thorax to groin region. Behaviour of most of the native dogs is more or less similar to terriers. In hot summer, free living dogs dig soil beneath shed for cooling the body. The digging is carried to excavate wet soil on which dog lies during the hot hours of the summer.

Classification of Domestic Dogs on the Basis of Utility

The domestic dogs have been classifies in different countries for fixing the standards of breeds by the Kennel Clubs. There is minor but ignorable differences in the standards of different countries. Since dog show competition is spreading and has become more or less international events, the standards are mutually adjusted in light of the standards of participating kennel clubs. The common classifications in vogue are the American classification and the British classification but in Europe, French and German classifications are also used in the respective countries. In this chapter, most of the known breeds have been listed in six categories of: (i) Breads of working Dogs or Non-Sporting Breeds, (ii) Utility Breeds, (iii) Terrier Breeds, (iv) Hound Breed (v) Gun Dogs and (vi) Toy Breeds.

I. Breeds of Working Dogs or Non-Sporting Breeds

1. Alaskan Malamute
2. Appenzell Mountain
3. Bearded Collie
4. Boxer
5. Beauceron
6. Briard (Berfer de Brie)

7. Bull Mastiff
8. Cane da Pastore
9. Cardigon Wlsh Corgi
10. Collie
11. Comondor
12. Cumberland Sheep Dog
13. Doberman Pinscher
14. Entlebuch Mountain Dog
15. Eskimo Dog
16. Fila Brasileiro
17. German Shepherd (Alsatian)
18. Great Dane
19. Great Swiss Mountain Dog
20. Groenendael
21. Hovawart
22. Karabash
23. Kuvasz
24. Landseer
25. Leonberger
26. Mastiff
27. Mastiff Espenol
28. Neopolitan Mastiff
29. New found land
30. Old English Sheep Dog
31. Penbroke Welsh Corgi
32. Puli
33. Pumi
34. Pyrenean Mastiff
35. Pyrenian Mountain Dog
36. Rottweiler
37. Saint Bernard
38. Shetland Shepherd Dog
39. Siberian Husky
40. South Russian Owtcharka

41. Swedish Vallhund
42. Tervueren
43. Tibetan Mastiff

II. Utility Breeds

1. Akita Inu
2. Boston Terrier
   a) Boston Terrier (Light weight)
   b) Boston Terrier (Medium weight)
   c) Boston Terrier (Heavy weight)
3. Chow Chow
4. Dalmation
5. Dogue de Bordeaux
6. Dunker
7. English Bull Dog
8. French Bull Dog
9. Lhasa Apso
10. Poodle, Standard
11. Poodle, Miniature
12. Poodle, Toy
13. Portuguese Shepherd Dog
14. Schnauzer, Giant
15. Schnauzer, Standard
16. Schnauzer, Miniature
17. Shar Pei
18. Shih Tzu
19. Tibetan Terrier

III. Terrier Breeds

1. Airedale Terrier
2. Bedlington Terrier
3. Black Terrier (Russian Terrier)
4. Bohemian Terrier

5. Border Terrier
6. Bull Terrier
7. Cairn Terrier
8. Dandie Dinmont Terrier
9. Fox Terrier, smooth haired
10. Fox Terrier, wire haired
11. German Hunting Terrier
12. Glen Imaal Terrier
13. Irish Terrier
14. Kerry Blue Terrier
15. Lakeland Terrier
16. Manchester Terrier
17. Norfolk Terrier
18. Norwich Terrier
19. Otter Terrier
20. Scottish Terrier
21. Sealyham Terrier
22. Skye Terrier
23. Soft Coated Wheaten Terrier
24. Stafford Terrier
25. Welsh Terrier
26. West Highland White Terrier

IV. Hound Breeds

1. Afghan Hound
2. American Fox Hound
3. Azawakh
4. Bassenji, Forest Type
5. Bassenji, Savannah Type
6. Basset Hound
7. Basset Black Gaxogne
8. Basset Griffon Vendeen, Large Type

9. Basset Griffon Vendeen, Small type
10. Bavarian Schweisshund
11. Beagle
12. Blood Hound
13. Borzoi
14. Coon Hound
15. Dachshund, Standard smooth hair
16. Dachshund, Standard wire hair
17. Dachshund, Standard long hair
18. Dachshund, miniature smooth hair
19. Dachshund, miniature wire hair
20. Dachshund, miniature long hair
21. Deer Hound
22. Fox Hound
23. Galgo Spanol
24. Great German Spitz
25. Grey Hound
26. Hanoverian Schweisshund
27. Harrier
28. Ibizan Hound
29. Irish Wolf Hound
30. Italian Grey Hound
31. Magyar Agar
32. Hound Breed
33. Portuguese Hound, Large
34. Portuguese Hound, Medium
35. Portuguese Hound, Small
36. Rhodesian Ridgeback
37. Saluki
38. Sloughi
39. Small Spitz

40. Toy Spitz
41. Whippet
42. Wolf Spitz

V. Gun Dogs / Sporting Breeds

1. American Cocker Spaniel
2. American Water Spaniel
3. Chesapeake Bay Retriever
4. Clumber Spaniel
5. Curley Coat Retriever
6. Deutsch Stichelhaar
7. Drentse Patrijshond
8. English Cocker Spaniel
9. English Setter
10. English Springer Spaniel
11. Epagneul Brelton
12. Epagneul Francais
13. Epagneul Picard
14. Flat Coated Retriever
15. German Long Haired Pointer
16. German Short Haired Pointer
17. German Wire Haired Pointer
18. German Spaniel
19. Golden Retriever
20. Gorden Setter
21. Hungarian Vizsla
22. Irish Setter
23. Irish Spaniel
24. Labrador Retriever
25. Munsterlander, Large
26. Munsterlander, Small

27. Perdigueiro de Burgos
28. Perdigueiro Portugues
29. Pointer
30. Poodle Pointer
31. Spinone
32. Sussex Spaniel
33. Weimaraner
34. Welsh Springer Spaniel
35. Wetter Hund

VI. Toy Breeds

1. Affenpinscher
2. Australian Terrier
3. Bichon Frise
4. Brabancon
5. Cavaliar King Charles Spaniel
6. Chihuahua
7. Chinese Crested Dog
8. English Toy Terrier
9. Griffon Belge
10. Griffon Bruxellois
11. Harlequin Pinscher
12. Japanese Chin (Japanese Spniel)
13. King Charles Spaniel
14. Lowchen
15. Maltese
16. Mexican Hairless
17. Miniature Pinscher
18. Pekingese
19. Pug
20. Silky Terrier

21. Tibetan Terrier
22. Yorkshire Terrier

2.4 Some Lesser Known and Recent Developed Breeds

1. Alaskan Klee Kai
2. Argentina Dogo
3. Barbet
4. Basset Fauve
5. Berger des Pyrenees
6. Bosanski
7. Brazilian Mastiff
8. Brazilian Terrier
9. Miniature Siberian Husky
10. Peruvian Hairless Dog
11. Elo
12. Thai Bangkaew Dog
13. Kangal Turkish Dog
14. Akbas Turkish Dog
15. American Hairless Terrier
16. Old English Bulldog (Old Bulldogge or Leavitt Bulldog)
17. Aussie Bulldog (Australian Bulldog)
18. Dorset Old Time Bulldog (Old Time Bulldog)
19. Tamaskan Dog
20. Shiloh Shepherd Dog
21. Lopo Italiano
22. Kunming Dog
23. Black Russian Terrier
24. Moscow Toy Terrier
25. Silken Windhound
26. Silken Windsprite

2.5 Some Indian Breeds of Dog

Domesticated Indian dogs are found in different shape and size. There are some good breeds evolved by local people for their regional utility. These are mostly refined native dogs of the area and a few have been evolved by cross breeding with one or more breeds of exotic dogs brought by nomads and travellers from the other countries. These are distributed from the high Himalayan region to coastal region. Indian domesticated dogs may be classified into following classes:

1. Working dogs: These may include Himalayan Sheep Dog, Bhutia, Gaddi, Dhangarhi and Tehri Bongara.
2. Hound group: This group includes Banjara, Chippiparai, Combai, Kucchi, Mahratha, Mudhol, Poligar, Rajapalayam, Rampur hound, Sindhi hound, Vanjari hound and Waghari.
3. Terrier group: Bhutia Bully, Sikkimese and Bhutanese.
4. Lesser known dogs of distinct features:
    a) Dogs of Himalayan region: Bongara Mastiff of Tehri Garhwal; Bisben of middle Himalayan areas, Kinnaur sheep dog of Lahaol-Spiti and Vikhan sheep dog of Chitral.
    b) Dogs of North-East region: Tezpuri of Tezpur area, Tripuri or Lusai of Tripura and Lushai hills of Meghalaya.
    c) Dogs of South India: Alangu, Kachi of nomads, Kaikadi of Tanjavore and Pathi of Nomadic tribe of Tamil Nadu.

Many ancient Indian breeds could not survive due to change in society under the influence of European intruders causing drastic disturbances in social, cultural and economic status of the common people. A separate class developed under the influence of English empire imported European breeds and provided them patronase by establishing Kennel clubs and organizing Dog shows for pleasing English bosses. The another pity situation is the under mining of the intelligence, agility and ability of indigenous dogs without studying their performances for retrieving, guarding, searching, seizure and guiding, etc.

2.6 Brief Description of Dog Breeds of Different Classes

A. Working Breeds

This group includes multipurpose breeds evolved in Europe and USA by cross breeding and rigorous selection using germplasm of several breeds.

1. **Alaskan Malamute**: It is a refined form of Siberian Husky brought by Eskimos during their translocation to Alaskan area of Arctic zone in Canada. Height of dog at shoulders is 64-71 cm and that of bitch is 58-66 cm; and body weight range is 38-56 kg, the males being larger. Facemask is essential. Coat colour ranges from greish black to black with greyish white ventral aspect from jowl to vent. Feathered tail is carried high but not coiled. (Fig.2.7)

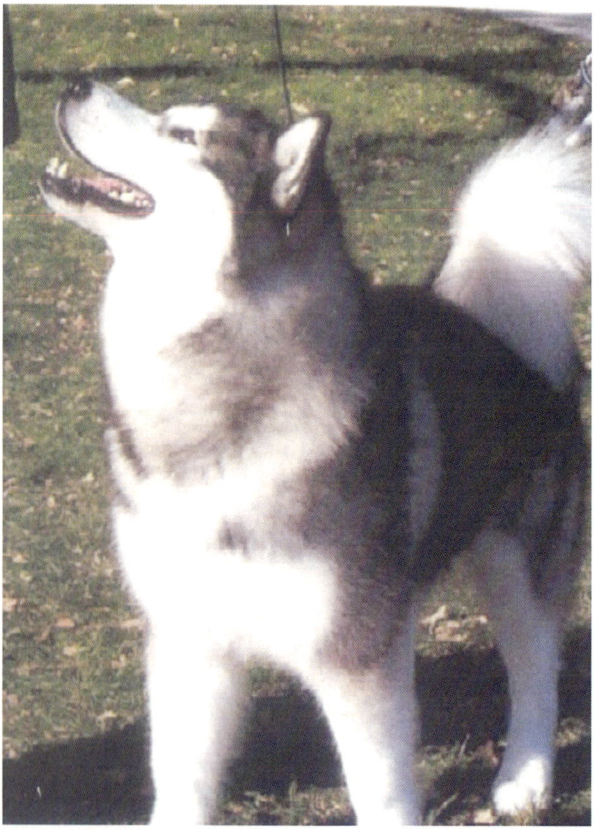

Fig. 2.7 Alaskan Malamute

2. **Briard:** The dog is handsome and docile French breed. Height: dog, 62-68 cm and bitch, 56-64 cm. Weight is not standardized. Coat is all solid colours except the white. Ears are pricked and tail is moderate with shallow upward turning of distal end. Limbs are boned.

3. **Beauceron or Berger de Beauce:** It is a hairy breed with fully feathered tail. Ear flaps are dropped. Face is short and covered with long hairs. Height: dog, 60-70 cm and bitch, 58-68 cm; weight, 27-37 kg, males are heavier.

4. **Boxer:** It is a composite German breed. Height at shoulders for dog is 57-63 cm and bitch 53-59 cm. Body weight of dog is 30-32 kg and bitch 25-27 kg. It possesses a dark mask. Coat colour is mostly brindle, reddish brown, pale fawn and fawn white. Ears are dropped at birth but mostly cropped to make prick. (Fig.2.8)

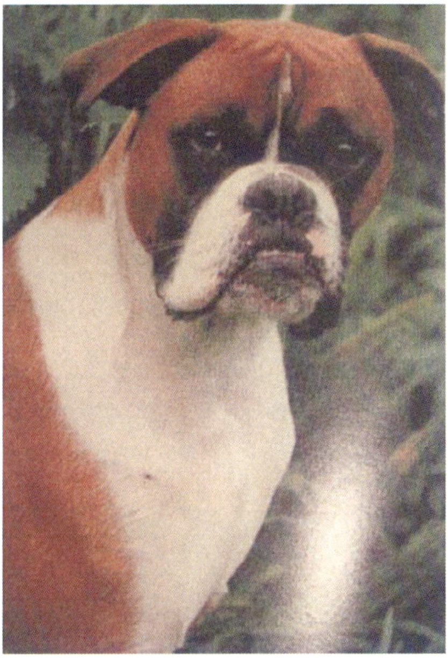

Fig. 2.8 Boxer

5. **Bull Mastiff**: It ia a large sized dog of strong frame, broad head, and short muzzle. Dropped medium size ears are placed apart on the skull. Height at shoulders of dog is 63.5-68.5 cm and bitch is 61-66 cm. Body weight of dog is 50-59 kg and bitch is 41-54 kg. Coat is short, dense, hard and smooth, and colour is any shade of brindle, red or fawn. (Fig.2.9)

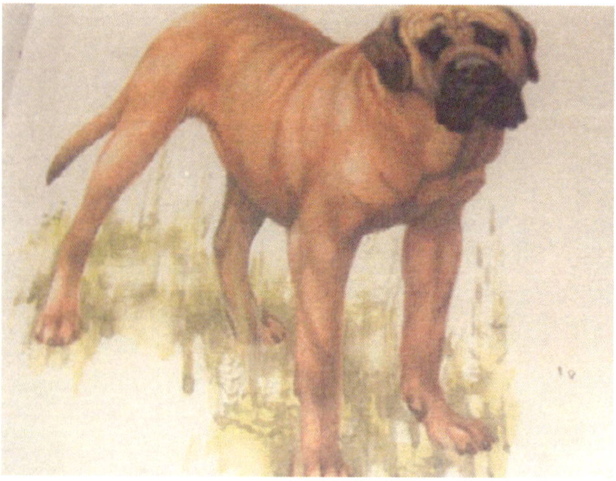

Fig. 2.9 Bull Mastiff

6. **Collie**: It is handsome, intelligent, trainable, agile and faithful sheep dog. Height at shoulders of dog is 56-61 cm and bitch is 51-56 cm with body weight 20.5-29.5 kg. Coat colour is sable and white, tricolour or blue merle. Coat may be long haired or short haired. Erect ears bend at the tip. Face is narrower. (Fig.2.10)

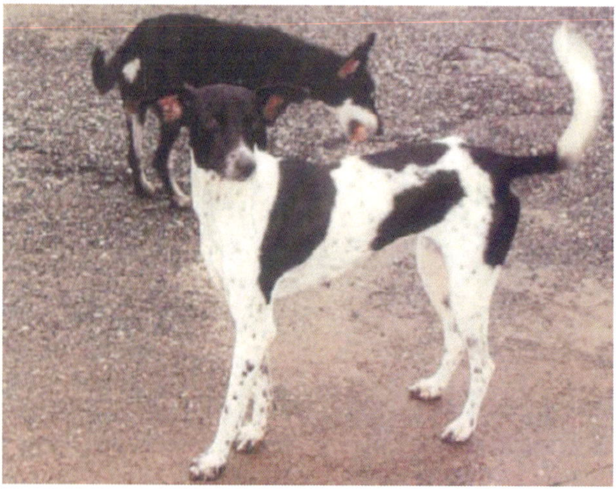

Fig. 2.10 Collie

7. **Dobermann Pinscher**: It is an intelligent, powerful, obedient and hardy. Height at shoulders is, dog 66-71 cm and bitch 61-66 cm; and body weight 30-40 kg. Coat colour is black, brown, fawn or blue. Limbs are bonned and muzzle is long. (Fig.2.11)

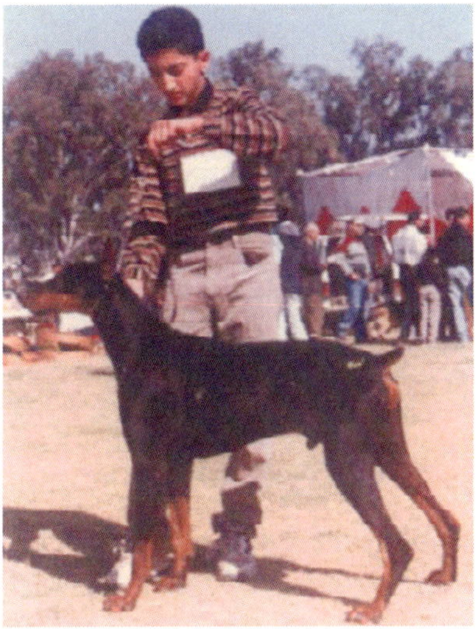

Fig. 2.11 Dobermann Pinscher

8. **German Shepherd or Alsatian**: Generally, three types of dogs are found. The differences are small and mainly in body coat which may be: (i) short, hard and close to body, (ii) longer coat with slightly wire hair and (iii) long haired . Height of dog is 62-66 cm and bitch is 51-55 cm, and deviations on either end are not accepted. Body weight range is 35 to 38.6 kg (77-85 lb). Coat is mostly wolf colour but may be black grey, steel grey or ash grey. It is one of the popular multipurpose dog used for guarding in different services.(Fig.2.12)

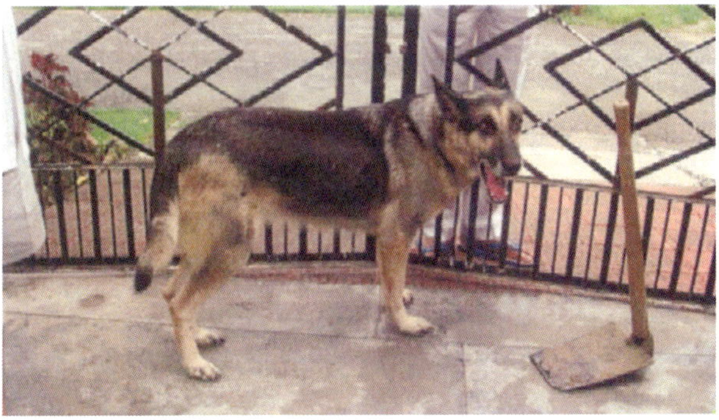

Fig. 2.12 German Shepherd / Alsatian

9. **Great Dane**: It is a graceful tall dog of lighter frame. The dog is intelligent, agile and loyal. Natural ears are flapped and made erect by surgery.Coat is short and smooth, and colour may be

brindle, brown, fawn or white ground with blue or black spots. Height: dog, 76-90 cm; bitch, below 71 cm. Body weight: dog, 54 kg and bitch,46 kg. (Fig.2.13)

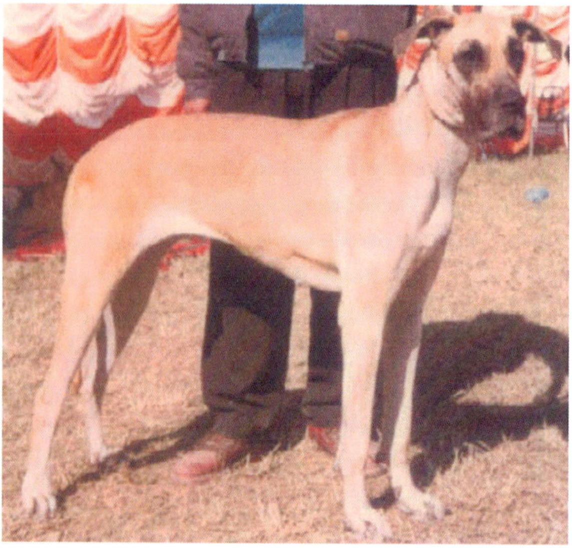

Fig. 2.13 Great Dane

10. **Groendael:** It is a Belgian shepherd dog evolved by selective breeding of a native dog of south Brussels. It is a long limbed slender dog covered with dense and smooth coat of long hairs. The dog is very sensitive and requires gentle handing. Height at withers: dog,61-66 cm; bitch, 56-61 cm; and body weight 28-35 kg. Coat colour is mostly solid black or black with white spots on feet and chest.

11. **Hovawart:** It is developed from the native dog of Black forest and high lands of central Germany. It is a multipurpose dog of calm and good nature friendly with children but fierce with intruders and enemies. Height at withers; dog,63-70 cm and bitch, 58-65 cm; body weight, dog, 30-40 kg and bitch, 25-35 kg. Coat colour may be black, deep black without white hairs or whole colour golden yellow. Long tail is bushy and medium ears are dropped.

12. **Leonberger**: A German tall and heavy breed. It is a lion like dog of pleasing disposition, docile and friendly with children. Despite of large size, the dog is very active. Height at shoulders; dog, 72-80 cm and bitch,65-76 cm; Weight 60-80 kg. Coat is lion colour,

golden yellow or brownish yellow with dark mask. Medium size ears are dropped. Underside colour may be slightly faint.

13. **Karabash:** It is an Anatolian ancient shepherd dog of Turkey. The body is heavily feathered and medium ear flaps are dropped. Face mask is darker. Coat colour is cream to golden brown. Height; dog, 74-81 cm and bitch, 71-79 cm. Body weight of dog is 50-64 kg and that of bitch is 41-59 kg.

14. **Mastiff:** It is an ancient European dog of large size that was used initially in wars and later on for hunting large game. The skin is wrinkled and coat is short, dense and smooth. It is a gentle dog of good nature only to known persons and other subjects. Minimum height 75 cm and weight 75-90 kg or even more. Approximate body weight can be worked out at the rate of 1 kg per cm height. Coat colour may be all shades of fawn, apricosa, silver or brindle. (Fig.2.14)

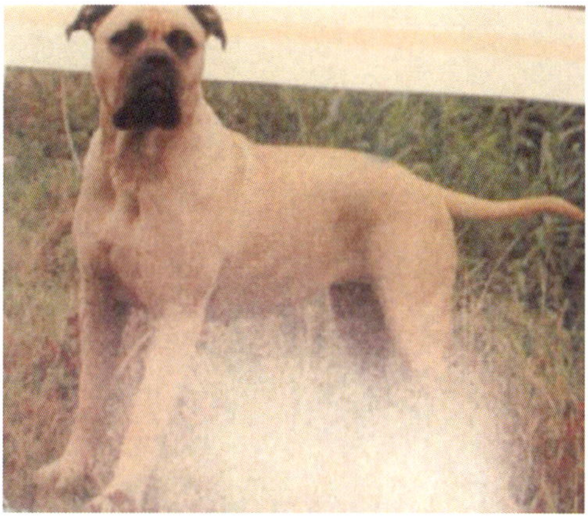

Fig. 2.14 Mastiff

15. **Mastiff Espenol or Spanish Mastiff**: It is a large dog of Spain. The dog is gentle and friendly particularly with children and aggressive towards strangers, unknown dogs and other animals. It is lighter than the English Mastiff. Height at withers; dog, 65-71 cm and bitch 67 cm. Body weight may be 50-60 kg. Coar colour is golden yellow, reddish brown and white with golden yellow or red patches.

16. **Neapolitan Mastiff**: It is an ancient fighting dog of Roman period. Behaviour of dog is variable and mostly depends on the training and strain. Some dogs are gentle and obedient while

some others do not care for commands. Height at withers; dog, 65-75 cm and bitch 65-70 cm; and body weight 60-70 kg. Coat colour is black, brown, brindle or lead grey. White markings are accepted on breast and toes.

17. **New found land**: It is a good retriever and effective workforce in water. It is used for rescuing drowning person due to its strength and swimming ability. Height at withers; dog, 71 cm and bitch 65 cm. Adult body weight of dog 64-69 kg and bitch 50-54.5 kg. Coat is thick, coarse and close to body; and coat colour is dark black. Tail is heavily feathered. Fringed ears are dropped on sides.

18. **South Russian Owtcharka**: It is a cross between Spanish and Tartar breed of Russia. It is a reliable shepherd dog. Height is 62-65 cm and body weight 35-40 kg. Coat colour may be white, yellowish white, spotted ash grey or bluish white due to a grey undercoat.

19. **Pyrenean Mastiff**: It is a massive Hungarian working dog. It is intelligent, brave, obedient and cordial with children. Heavy coat covering around the body requires daily combing for preventing mat formation on ears, around vent and external genitalia. Height; dog 70-81 cm and bitch 65-73.5; weight 45-55 kg. The outer coat is thick, moderately long and straight and undercoat is fine woolly. Colour may be white, badger colour, wolf grey patches on ears, head and base of the tail.

20. **Rottweiler**: It is a German breed developed for driving cattle and guarding households and yards. It is a good natured dog, interested in retrieving and eager track follower. It is a dominant breed and needs firm hand for controlling. Its bite is firm and attacks without warning. Height; dog 63-69 cm and bitch 58-63.5 cm; and body weight around 35 kg. Coat colour is black with tan shades on sides of face, chest and distal and parietal aspects of legs, nose and lips are definitely black. The ears are dropped and stop is deep. (Fig.2.15)

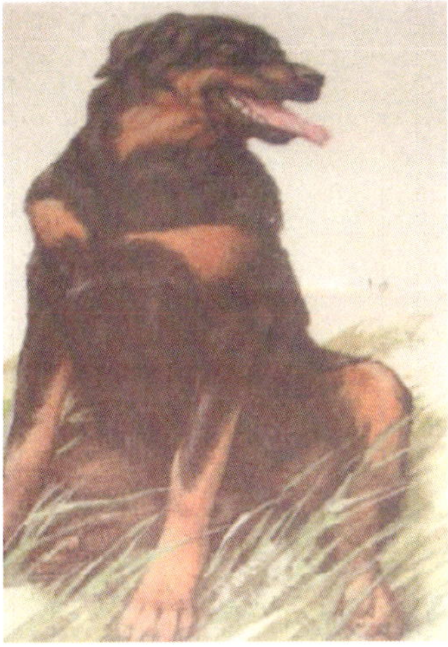

Fig. 2.15 Rottweiler

21. **Saint Bernard**: It is a dog of Alps mountain. It is an excellent rescue dog quiet, friendly and devoted to master. A trained dog can search a person from long distance in a snow covered area. Height; dog, minimum 75 cm and bitch, minimum 70 cm. Body weight; dog 80-85 kg and bitch 75-78 kg. Head is broad and muzzle is short. The colour is pure red and white with white blaze, collar, muzzle, breast, belly, legs and tip of the tail. Body is covered with long coat and tail is feathered. Ear flaps drop on either side.(Fig.2.16).

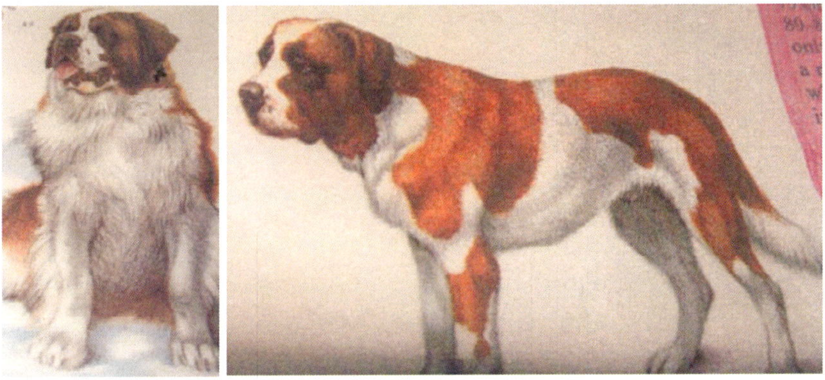

Fig. 2.16 Saint Bernard

22. **Samoyed**: It is working breed of Arctic region used for pulling sladge on snow and assistance in hunting. It is a member of spitz group. The compact body is covered with double coat- a thick,

soft and woolly undercoat covered with outer coat of long coarse hairs. The almond shaped eyes are dark and bright. Nose may be black, brown or liver colours compact square body is carried on bonds limbs. Tail is feathered and coiled. Prick ears face forward and their under surface is clean. White coat colour is preferred but may be yellowish white, off white or white and yellow. (Fig.2.17)

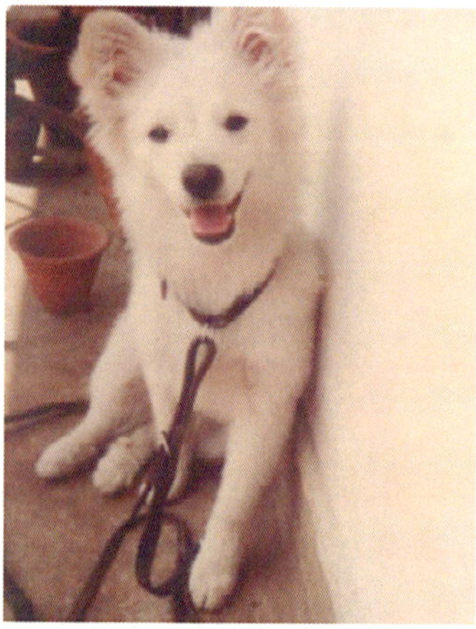

Fig. 2.17 Samoyed

B. Utility Breeds

1. **Boston Terrier**: It is an amiable, intelligent, playful, courageous and faithful companion. Ears are erect and muzzle is short. Height 35-45 cm and body weight less than 11.5 kg. This breed is further differentiated into three types on the basis of body weight, i.e: (i) light weight less than 6.8 kg, (ii) middle weight 6.9-9.0 kg and (iii) heavy weight 9.1-11.5 kg. Coat colour is brindle or black with white nose, blaze, jowl, breast, collar and legs. (Fig.2.18)

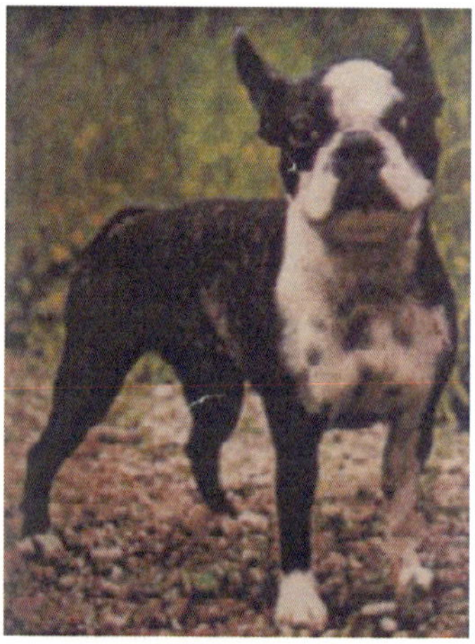

Fig. 2.18 Boston Terrier

2. **Chow Chow**: It is an ancient breed of China. It was reared for hunting and soft fur. Height of dog is 48-56 cm and that of bitch is 46-51 cm; and body weight range is 18-25 kg. Coat colour may be red, orange, fawn, blue, cream and white. (Fig.2.19)

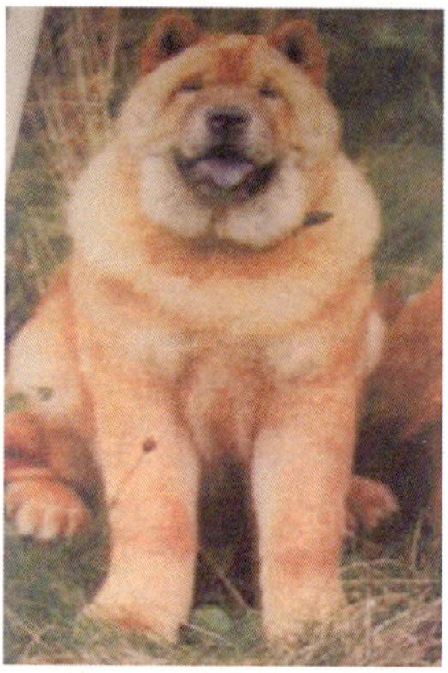

Fig. 2.19 Chow Chow

3. **Dalmation:** It is a dog of Asian origin refined by selective breeding in England. It is calm, docile and obedient. Height of dog is 58-61 cm and the bitch is 55.9-58.4 cm; and body weight 23-25 kg. Coat is white with well-defined black or tan spots irregularly distributed on the body. The spots on face, limbs and tail are smaller. Tapering tail bends upwards like a sickle. Muzzle is broader and ears are dropped. (Fig.2.20)

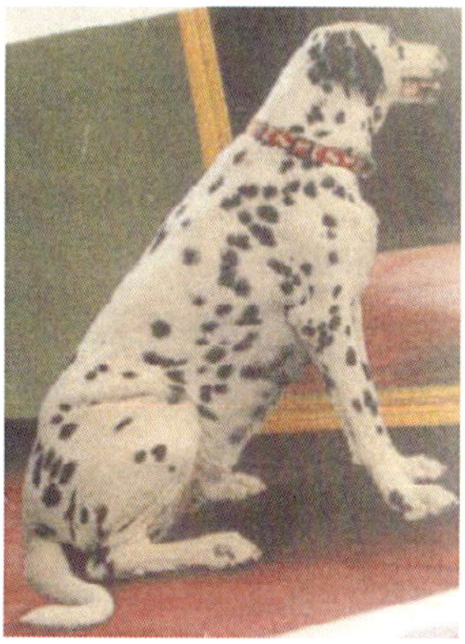

Fig. 2.20 Dalmation

4. **Dunker:** It is a leser known Norwegian breed lighter than the Dalmation. Height is 47-57 cm and weight is 18-20 kg. Coat colours are black, dark red and blue marbled. Few white markings are acceptable on marbled members. (Fig.2.21)

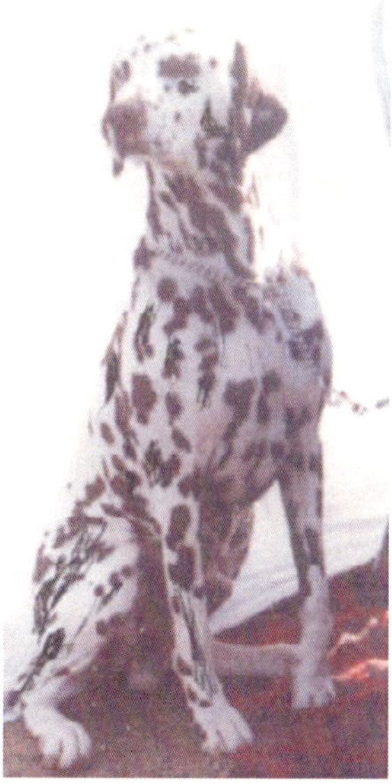

Fig. 2.21 Dunker

5. **English Bull dog**: It is an ancient English breed evolved for fight with bulls. It is a blocky dog with short, thick and deflected legs. Modern Bull dog is gentle, affectionate and intelligent. It does not require extensive exercise and can be kept in busy families also. Height is 40 cm and weight of dog is 25 kg and bitch 22.7 kg. The face is broad and wrinkled, muzzle is short and ears are half bent. The arms are a little arched due to which lion is higher than the shoulders. All colours except black, black and tan, black and white are accepted. A dark mask is present in the dogs of solid colour. (Fig.2.22)

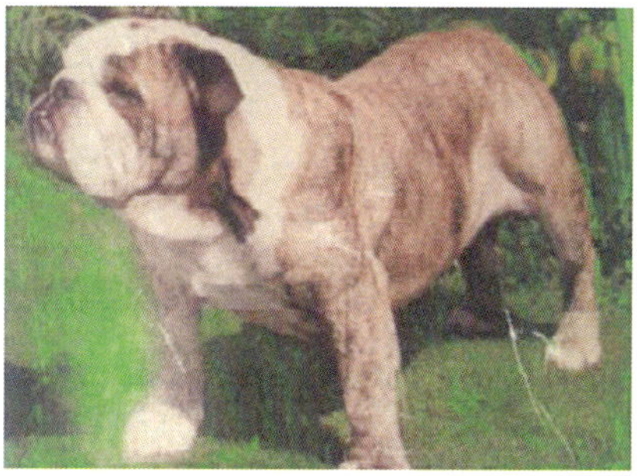

Fig. 2.22 English Bull dog

6. **French Bull dog:** It is an agile, intelligent and amiable dog which likes the company of children. Height 25-34 cm and body weight of dog 12-17 kg and that of bitch is 10.9 kg. Coat colour is brincle, brindle spots or patches on white ground and fawn may have brindle hairs. Pricked ears, short muzzle and wrinkled skin. Limbs are short and less arched than the English Bull dog.
7. **Lhasa Apso:** It is highly feathered double coated dog of Lhasa. Height is 25.5 cm and weight is 5-7 kg. Coat colour may be golden, fawn, sandy, slate grey or dark brown. (Fig.2.23)

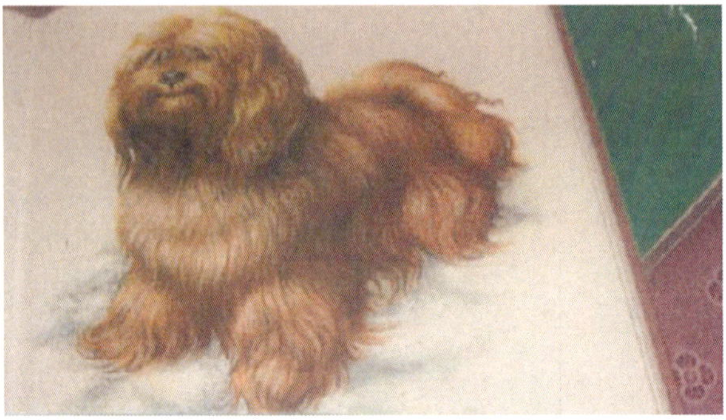

Fig. 2.23 Lhasa Apso

8. **Shih Tzu:** It is a double coated Chinese breed covered in profuse long hairs sweeping the ground. All colour coat is found but tip of the tail is white. (Fig.2.24)

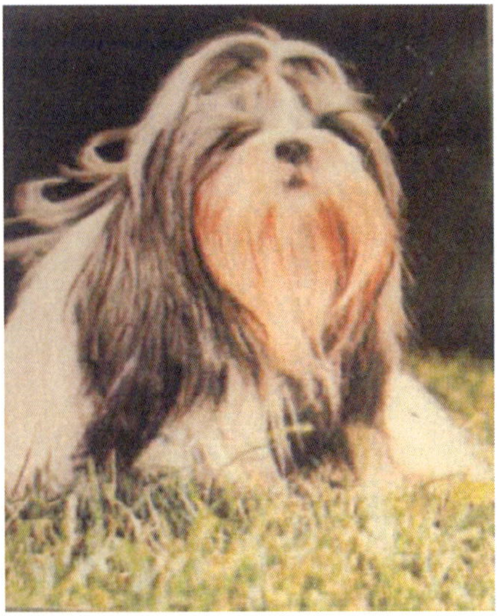

Fig. 2.24 Shih Tzu

C. Terrier Breeds

1. **Airedale Terrier:** It is a smart dog with long and flat skull, half dropped ears, small and dark eyes, hard wiry body coat of tan with black or dark grizle colour. Height at withers; dog 58.4-61 cm and bitch 55.9-58.4 cm; and body weight 20 kg. Ears are half bent V-shaped. (Fig.2.25)

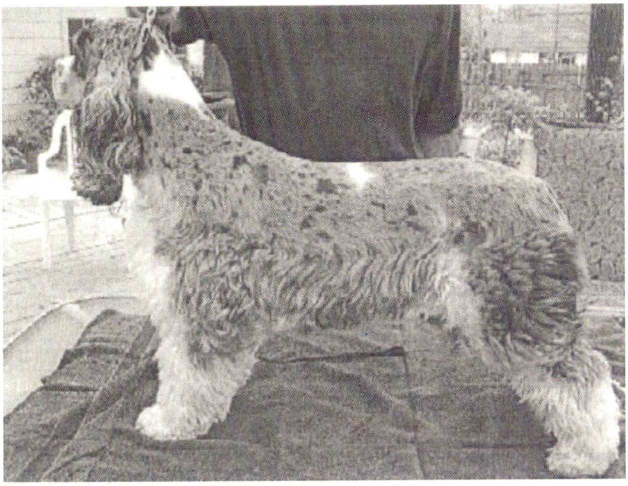

Fig. 2.25 Airedale Terrier

2. **Black Russian Terrier**: It is a Russian dog developed for military services. It is greater blood of Airedale Terrier. Height at shoulders of dog 66-72 cm and that of bitch 64-70 cm. Body weight about 40 kg. Coat colour is grey tinged black. Ears are dropped and stop is rudimentary. (Fig.2.26)

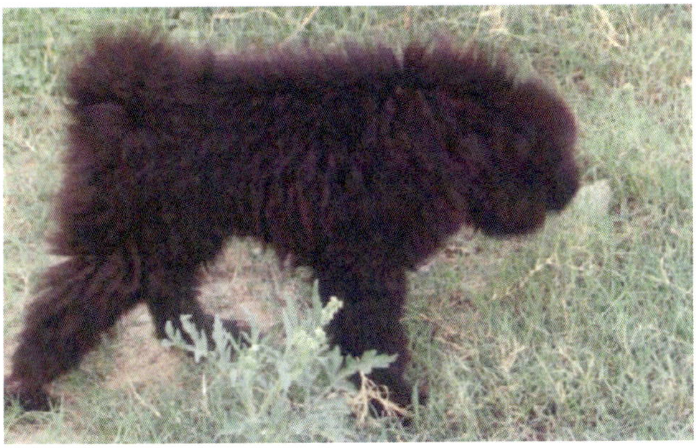

Fig. 2.26 Black Russion Terrier

3. **Bull Terrier**: It is a synthetic breed evolved for fighting. The dog is agile, faithful and very good companion. There is no standard for height or weight but for practical purpose height is 40-55 cm and body weight is 20-30 kg. Coat is short and dense, and colour is pure white with marking only on head or brindle. (Fig.2.27)

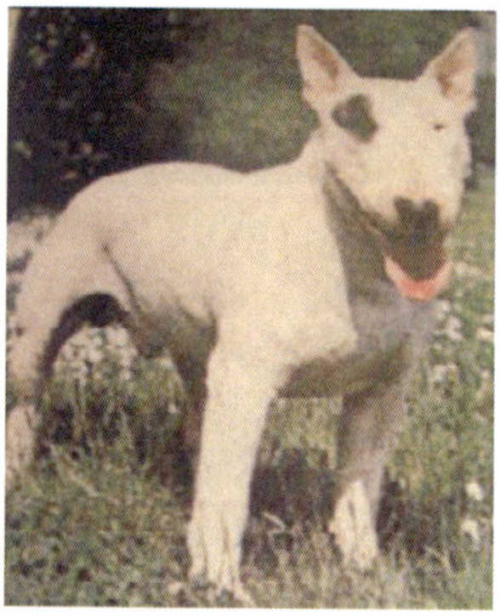

Fig. 2.27 Bull Terrier

4. **Fox Terrier**: It is developed as an excellent game dog. It is obedient, active, can work in water also but temperamental and unfit in house. Height, dog, less than 39.5 cm and bitch should be smaller. Body weight, dog 8.25 kg and bitch kg. Coat may be smooth haired or wire haired. Colour is not much important but may be brindle, liver or slate grey. (Fig.2.28)

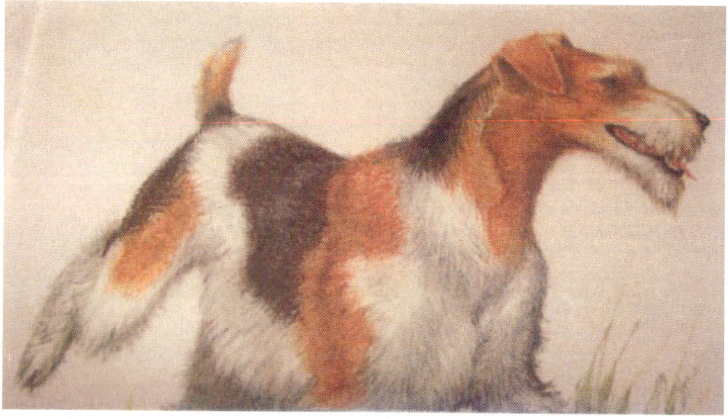

Fig. 2.28 Fox Terrier

5. **Manchester Terrier**: It is an active and playful dog good for companion and guarding. Height, dog 40-41 cm, bitch about 38 cm; weight 4-8 kg. Coat colour is black with tan shade on muzzle and limbs. Ears are half dropped. The tail is smooth and tapering in the form of upward turn sallow sickle.

6. **English Toy Terrier**: It is a miniature terrier of pleasing disposition. The dog is very active, energetic and playful. Height 25-30 cm, lower is better; and weight 2.7-3.6 kg. Coat colour is

tan black with white streaks on muzzle and an almost oval spot above the upper eyelids. Moderate prick ears are forward facing. (Fig.2.29)

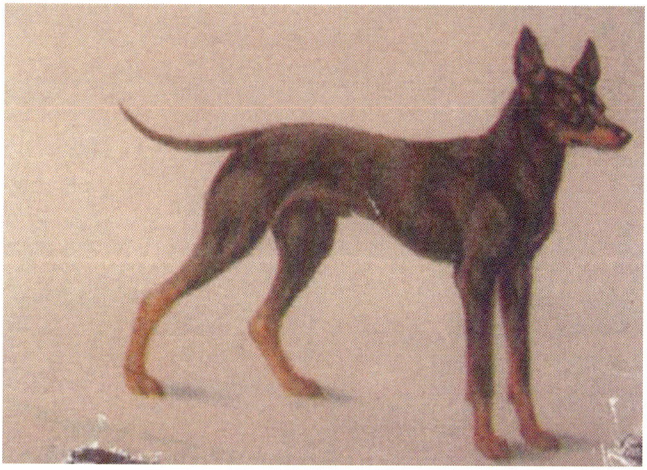

Fig. 2.29 English Toy Terrier

D. Hound Breeds

1. **Afghan Hound:** This magnificent breed is a native of Afghanistan. It is a tall, slender and well-feathered aristocritic dog. The head is long, straight and free from feathering. Height, dog 68.6-73.6 cm and bitch 61-68.6 cm; weight 25-30 kg. Coat colour; yellow brown with a dark mask, tan, dull red, greyish tan. (Fig.2.30)

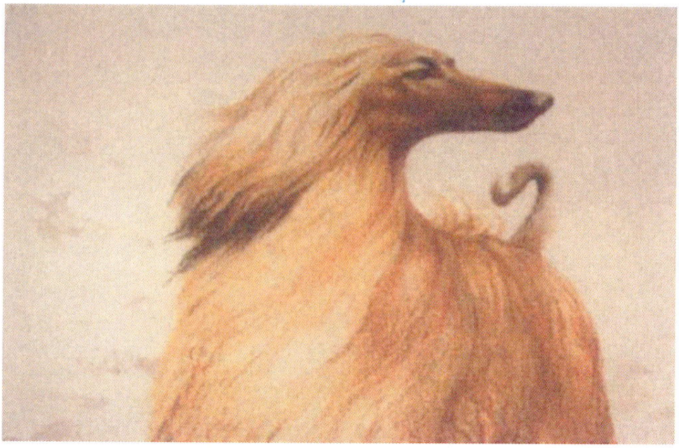

Fig. 2.30 Afghan Hound

2. **Bassenji:** It is a gun dog developed for hunting. Height, 40-43 cm and body weight 9-11 kg. Coat colour may be black, tan or chestnut with white patch on chest extending to form complete or broken collar. The tail is coiled on the back. (Fig.2.31)

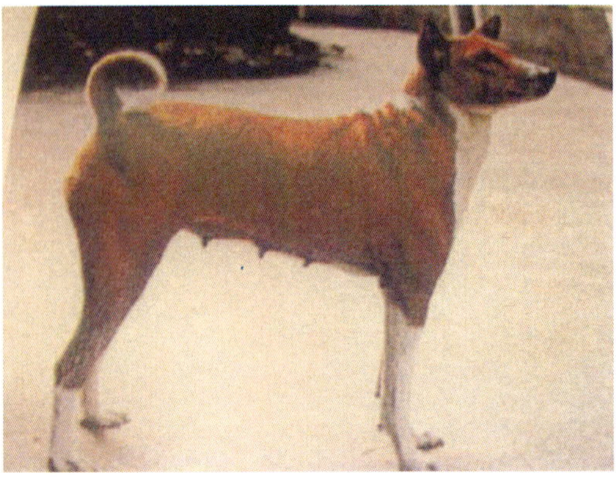

Fig. 2.31 Bassenji

3. **Basset Hound:** It is a short-legged, stumpy dog of compact body. Bones are heavy and strong. Ear flaps are very long, fleshy, dropped and reach below the level of throat. Height, 33-38 cm and weight 23 kg. Coat colour all types for recognized colour of hound and placement of markings on the body does not have any definite pattern. (Fig.2.32)

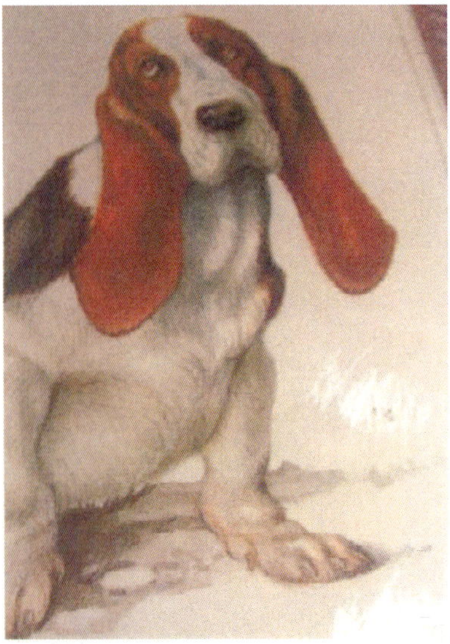

Fig. 2.32 Basset Hound

4. **Beagle**: The Beagle is a docile, gentle and peace loving dog. Handling of dog is very easy and it is a suitable companion and a house dog. Height is 33-40 cm and body weight is variable. Coat colour may be solid or liver colour with white patches of variable size. Diatal part of whip like tapering tail is always white and V-shape dropped ears are broad at base. (Fig.2.33)

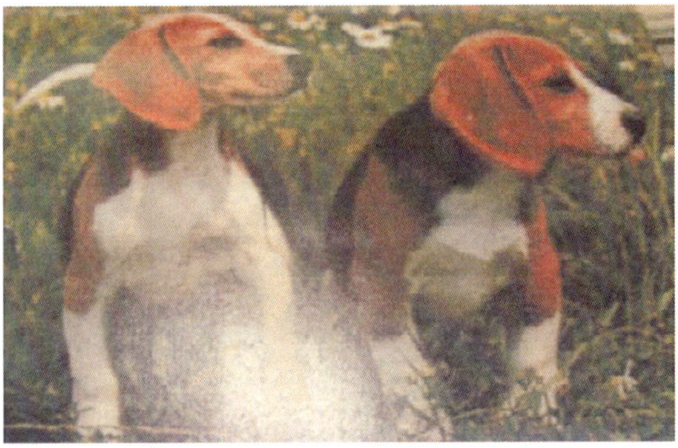

Fig. 2.33 Beagle

5. **Blood Hound**: It is a large breed of active habit but peace loving. Coat is short, dense and smooth. Coat colour may be mahogany red, black and tan or liver with black muzzle. Tapering stern tail and very large dropped ears.

6. **Borzoi:** It is a tall feathered dog with clean and narrow face and fringed dropped ears. Height, dog 74 cm and bitch 68 cm, and larger size is preferred. Body weight is 35-45 kg. Coat colour may be white with red, orange, yellow or brindle or grey patched. (Fig.2.34)

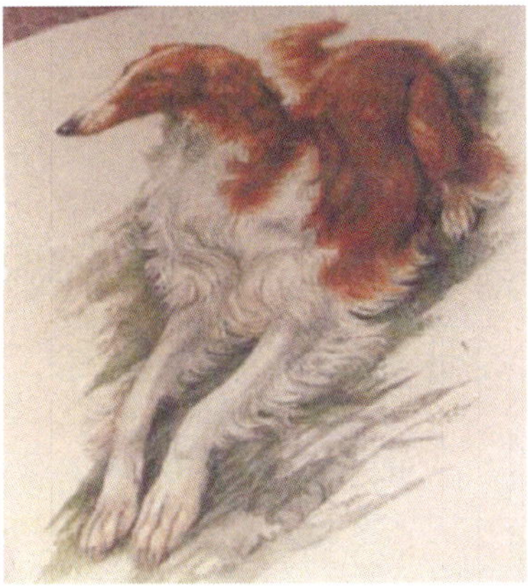

Fig. 2.34 Borzoi

7. **Dachshund**: A very short-legged dog of long body and tapering stern tail. Body coat may be short and smooth or straight long haired or wire haired. Height 20-25 cm and body weight of dog below 11.5 kg and bitch below 10.4 kg. Body weight of miniature type ranges from 4.5 to 5 kg. Colour is variable and almost all colours except solid black and white are accepted. (Fig.2.35)

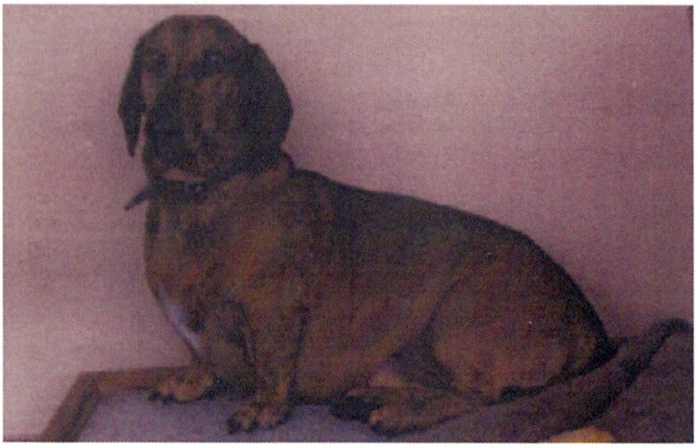

Fig. 2.35 Dachshund

8. **Grey Hound**: It is a tall, slender breed of light frame. Four legs are boned and straight and hind legs are angled to facilitate fast run. Height, dog 71-76 cm and bitch 68-71 cm, body weight 20-25 kg. Stomach is tucked up and moderate ears are dropped. Coat colour is variable, whole colour or patched. This dog requires extensive exercise. This breed is suitable for hunting and working at farms. It is not suitable for house and flats. (Fig.2.36)

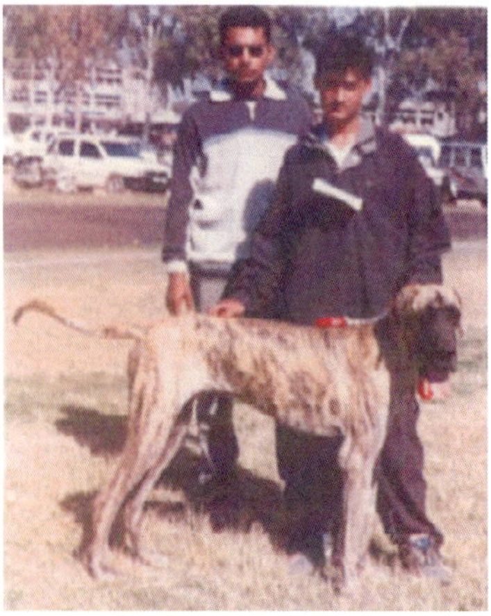

Fig. 2.36 Grey Hound

9. **Azawakh**: It is refined breed of slender and tall hounds of light frame and square structure. Head is long with narrow muzzle and dropped medium size ears. Croup is moderately sloppy and abdomen is tucked up. Coat colour ranges from sandy,yellowish red to red with black mask. It may also be brindle often with white markings on head, breast and tip of the long tail. Tail is tapering and bent upwards in the shape of a sickle. Height is about 70 cm and body weight upto 30 kg. This is a newer breed recognized and separated from Sloughi during 1981.

10. **Saluki**: It is a tall dog of light weight capable of fast run and capturing prey. The head is narrow with conical muzzle and posteriorly placed dropped ears. Tail bears flag like feathering. Height of dog is 58-71 cm and bitch 54-66 cm, and body weight 14-25 kg. Coat colour may be white, cream, fawn, golden yellow, golden red, black and tan, grey, grizzle, black with yellowish markings or combination of any of these colours. (Fig.2.37)

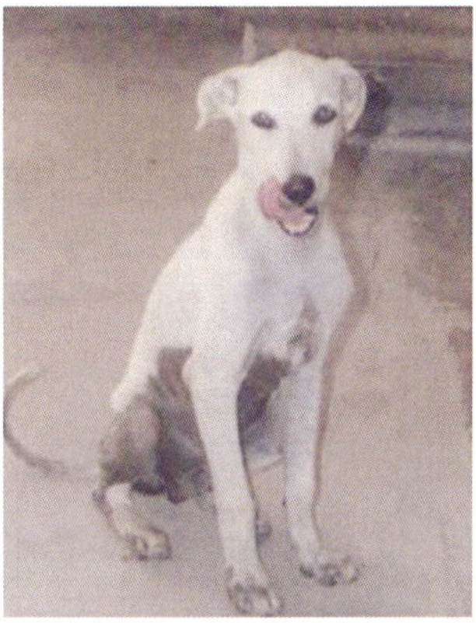

Fig. 2.37 Saluki

11. **Whippet**: It is more or less similar to Saluki group but much smaller in size. Height of dog is 47-51 cm and bitch 44-47 cm, and body weight 7.5-12 kg. Special feature is rose ear. Coat colour may be solid colour, mixed colour or brindle.

12. **Pomeranian :** It is one of the most common pet dog in India due to its active habits, sweet nature, small size, woolly body coat and bushy coiled tail. The ears are pricked, Nose is black, Eyes are small and situated at the level of stop. Body is coverd with the soft woolly under coat and long outer coat but face is free from long hairs. It belongs to spitz groups. The name has been derived from the place Pomerania, where it was developed to present form from the native Arctic region. The dog is obedient and like to play with children.Barks on strangers. Height is generally 30.5 c.m. or 12 inches and body weight 2-5 kg (4.4lb). Smaller specimens preferred. Common coat colour is white and others colours are (red, orange, fawn, lemon, etc.) should be free from shading. (Fig.2.38a,b)

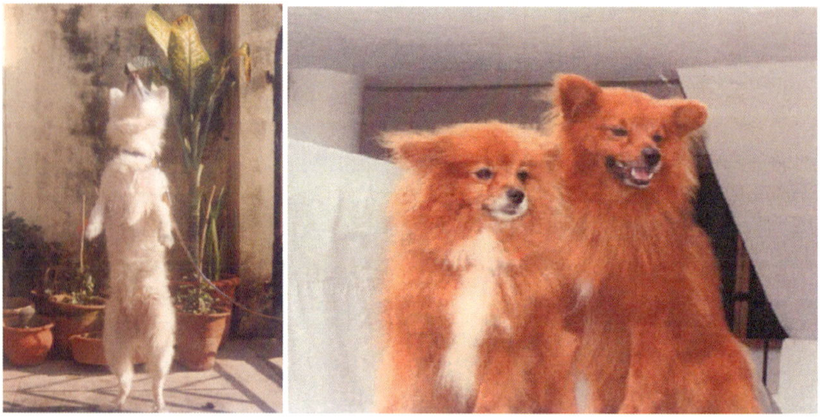

Fig. 2.38 Pomeranian

E. Gun Dogs or Hunting Dogs

1. **American Cocker Spaniel:** The original gun dog is now a companion pet. The body is covered with profuse long coat and very long drooping ears. Height of dog is 36.25-38.75 cm and bitch is 33.75-36.75 cm, body weight is 10-12 kg. Coat colour is whole colour black, red, golden or these may be with white patches. Some may be tricolour also. The head is short and broad with round crown. Muzzle is also short and broad.

2. **English Cocker Spaniel**: It is the parent of American Cocker Spaniel and both breeds are almost similar except that the English Cocker Spaniel is a little larger. Height is 38-41 cm and body weight range is 12.7-14.5 kg. (Fig.2.39)

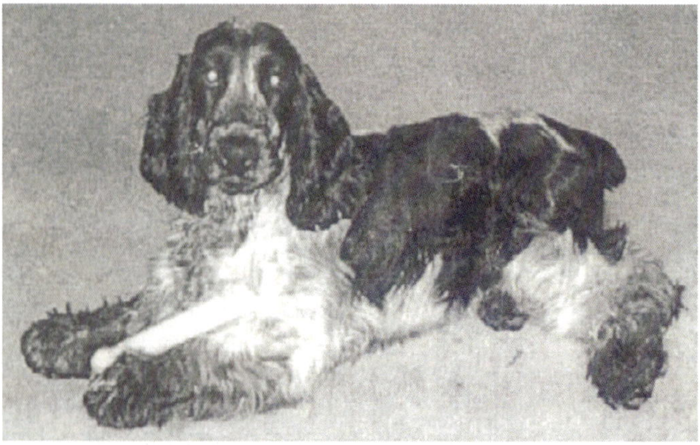

Fig. 2.39 English Cocker Spaniel

3. **English Setter**: It is an elegant and attractive dog of powerful compact body with stern tail. Ears hang in folds. Height at shoulders, dog 56.9-68.6 cm and bitch 53.3-64.8 cm, and body weight 27-32 kg. Coat colour black and white is more liked, and other colours are lemon and white, liver and white, tan and white. Small patches are preferred on white ground. (Fig.2.40)

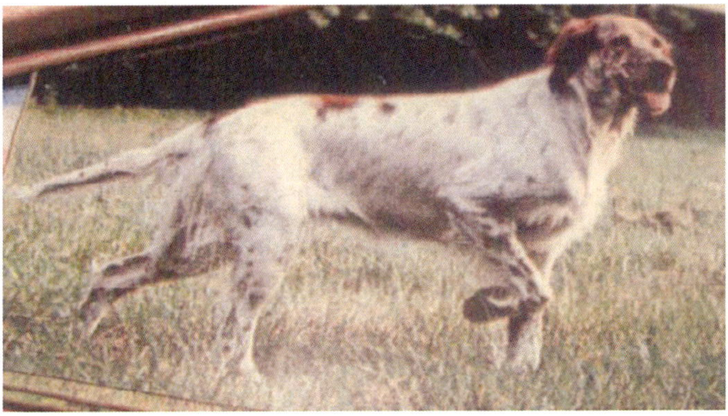

Fig. 2.40 English Setter

4. **German Pointer**: Three strains of this breed are short-haired, long-haired and wire-haired. Long ear flaps are dropped close to sides. Tail is feathered and limbs are bonned.

   a) **German Short Haired Pointer**: Height at shoulders, dog 58-64 cm and bitch 53-59 cm; and weight, dog 25-32 kg and bitch 20.5-27 kg. Colour, always liver head, body colour may be solid liver, liver with white marking on breast and legs or white with liver markings.

   b) **German Long Haired Pointer:** Coat colour is brown or white with brown markings and length of hairs is 3-5 cm but short at head.

   c) **German Wire Haired Pointer**: Height at withers of dog is 60-67cm and bitch 56-62 cm; weight of dog 25-34 kg and bitch 20.5-29 kg. Coat colour may be solid liver, liver and white or liver and black. Outer coat is curled, dense and coarse and dense undercoat lies close to body.

5. **Golden Retriever**: It is an active retriever with great indurance highly interested in water retrieving. It likes the company of children. Height, dog 56-61 cm and bitch 45-56 cm; and body

weight of dog 32-37 kg and bitch 27-32 kg. Coat colour may be all shades of golden without any pencling of red or tan. (Fig.2.41)

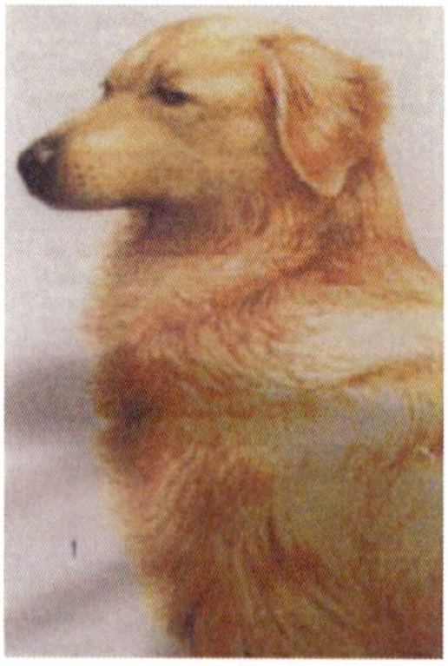

Fig. 2.41 Golden Retriever

6. **Labrador Retriever**: It is a short dog of compact body, bonned legs and strong neck. It is a hard working dog of indurence. Height, 56-57 cm and bitch 54-56 cm; and body weight 25-30 kg. Coat is short and dense and colour is solid black and different intensity of brown. (Fig.2.42)

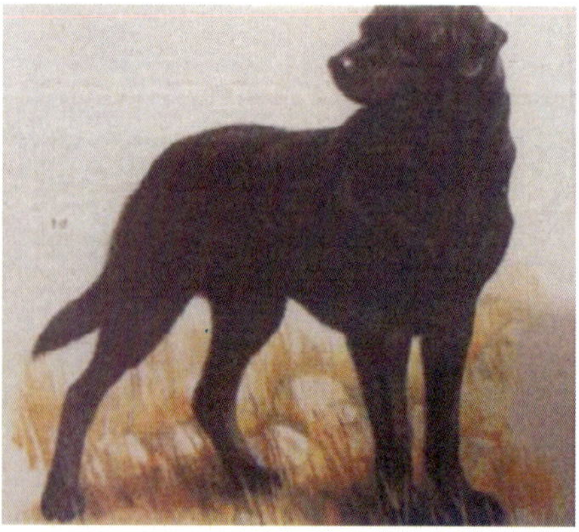

Fig. 2.41 Labrador Retriever

7. **Pointer**: It is an elegant dog of robust personality and majestic look. The large ears are dropped close to head. Smooth tail is like stern. Height, dog 63-69 cm and bitch 61-66 cm; and body weight 25-30 kg. Coat is short, dense and smooth, and colour may be white with yellow, orange or brown or black patches. Self-coloured dogs are also found. (Fig.2.43)

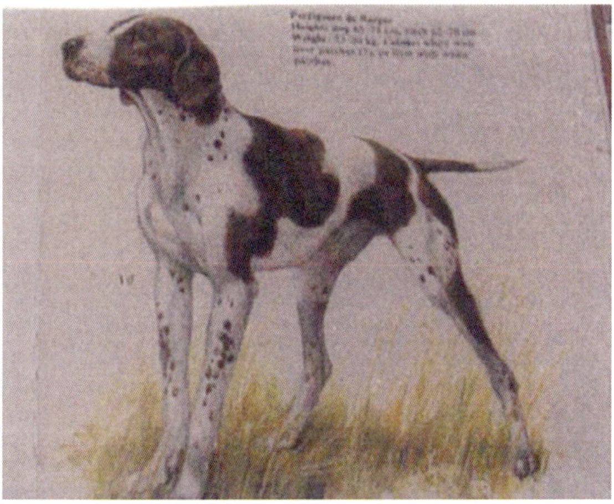

Fig. 2.43 Pointer

8. **Weimaraner:** It is a tall dog of light frame. The coat may be short and dense or long haired. Head is broad, jaws are flued and long ear flaps are dropped close to skull. Height of dog is 61-69 cm and bitch is 56-64 cm; and body weight 23-28 kg. Coat colour may be different shades of grey. There may be white marks on head and breast. Tail is feathered like flag in hairy type.

F. Toy Breeds

1. **Affenpinscher:** It is a beautiful tiny dog covered with long coat. The head is round, muzzle is short and short-legged. Height is 23 cm and body weight should not be more than 4 kg. The hairs on face are bristle like and undressed. It is an ancient German breed. (Fig.2.44)

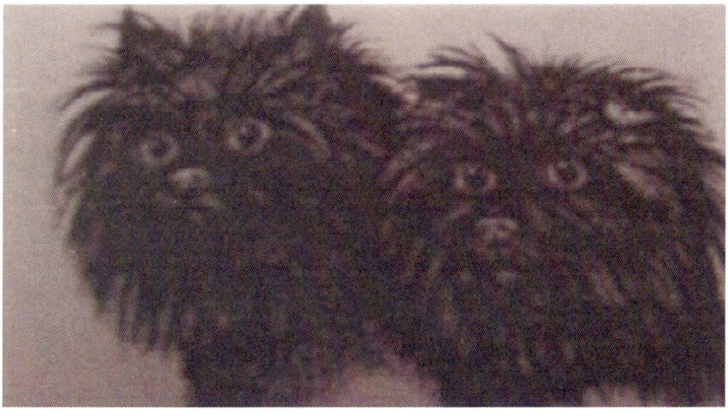

Fig. 2.44 Affen Pinscher

2. **Cavalier King Charles Spaniel:** It is a pleasant dog of active habits and sporting behaviour. The dark eyes are prominent and drooping long ears are set high on skull. Long silky coat is formed of freely hanging fine fibres with slight wavyness. The ears, legs and tail are fully feathered. Height 33.5-33 cm; and body weight 5.5-8.2 kg. Coat colour is black and tan, glossy black with mahogany mark on the forehead extending to anterior part of muzzle and also on the legs, white with chestnut red patches and characteristic style.
3. **Chihuahua**: It is probably the smallest dog on the earth. It may be short-haired or long-haired. Prick ears are placed apart and inclined sideward. Head is large and muzzle is short. Height 15-23 cm and body weight 0.9-2.7 kg and lighter is preferred. (Fig.2.45)

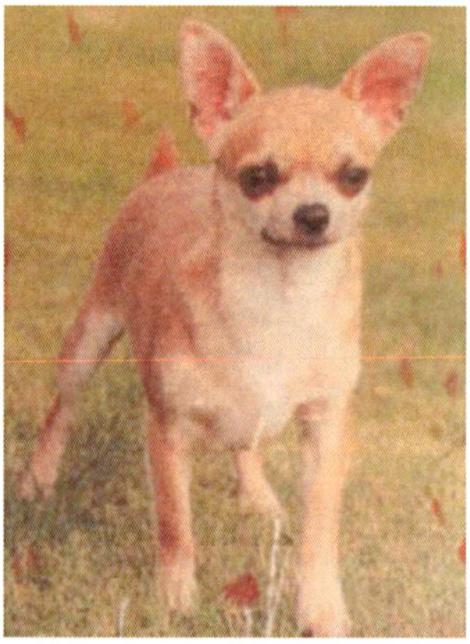

Fig. 2.45 Chihuahua

4. **Chinese Crested Dog**: This is a hairless breed with long hairs on head, distal part of legs and tip of the tail. Muzzle is short, eyes are bright and erect ears are fringed. Height 28-33 cm and weight below 5.5 kg. All coat colours are accepted. The breed has also been differentiated into deer type with long and slender legs and cobby type of short legs.
5. **Mexican Hairless Dog:** This is a breed of central Mexico because clay models of dog are found in the excavation of graves of Aztec people. This breed does not bark but whine and howl. Height may be about 30 cm and body weight below 5 kg. Any whole colour or patched colour is accepted but grey, pink or greyish-pink are common.

6. **Griffons Belge:** This is a lively guard dog of calm nature. Height is 21-28 cm and body weight 2.7-4.5 kg. Coat colour is black or with rusty markings.

7. **Griffon Bruxellois**: Same as Griffon Belge except coat colour is red or rusty with dark mask.

8. **Bichon Frise**: It is closely related to Maltese. At one time, it was the most preferred dog of French ladies. Height should not be more than 28 cm and body weight should be below 4 kg. Fully feathered coat is white but very light colour of ears is accepted. (Fig.2.46)

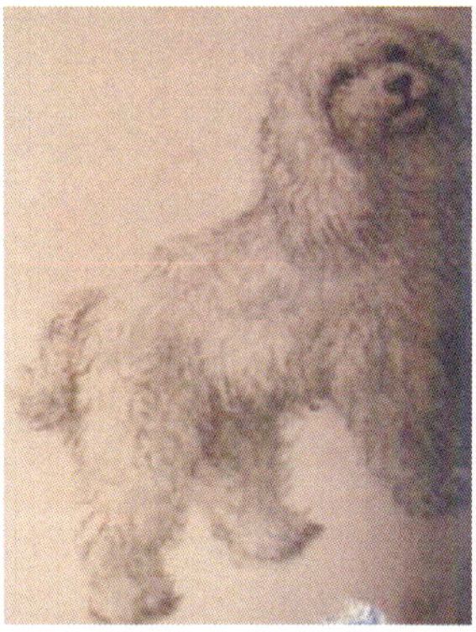

Fig. 2.46 Bichon Frise

9. **Lowchen:** The meaning is little lion dog. It is a rare breed. It's height at shoulders is 20-35 cm and body weight 2.5-3 kg. Coat colour should be preferably white, lemon or black, but other colours are allowed. Hair dressing in lion style is common. (Fig.2.47)

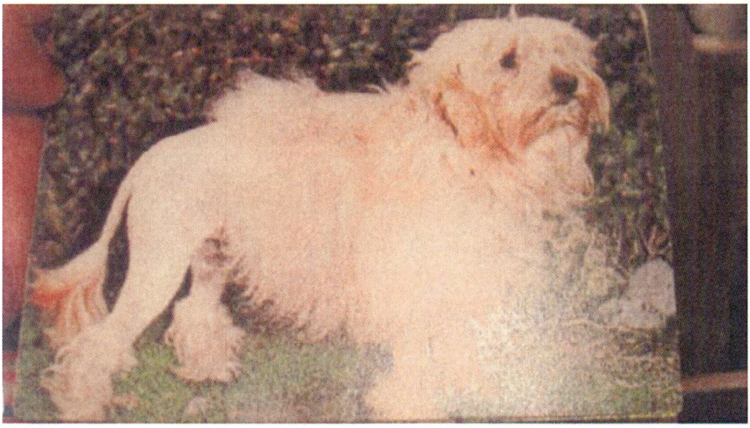

Fig. 2.47 Lowchen

10. **Maltese**: It is a native of Yuloslavia and has no link of origin in Malta island. It was pet of ladies of Rome and Athens. Height Less than 25.5 cm and body weight 3-4 kg. Coat colour is white and formed of long fur. (Fig.2.48)

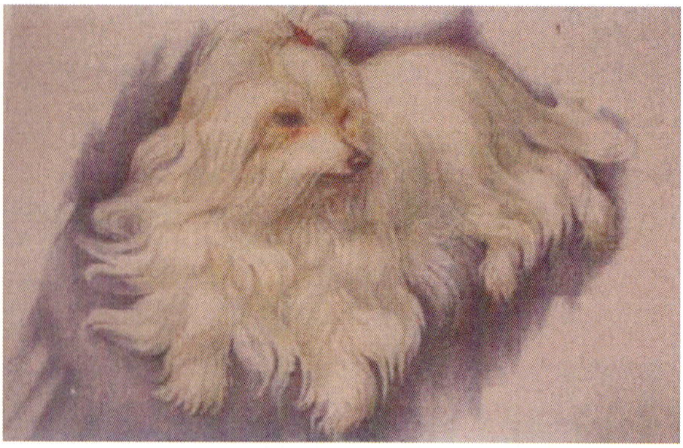

Fig. 2.48 Maltese

11. **Miniature Pinscher:** This oldest German breed was evolved by rigorous selection for evolving a tiny pinscher dog. It is an active and playful dog liked by the children. Height is 25-30 cm and body weight 3-4 kg. Coat colour may be reddish brown, black with tan and blue-grey with tan markings. (Fig.2.49)

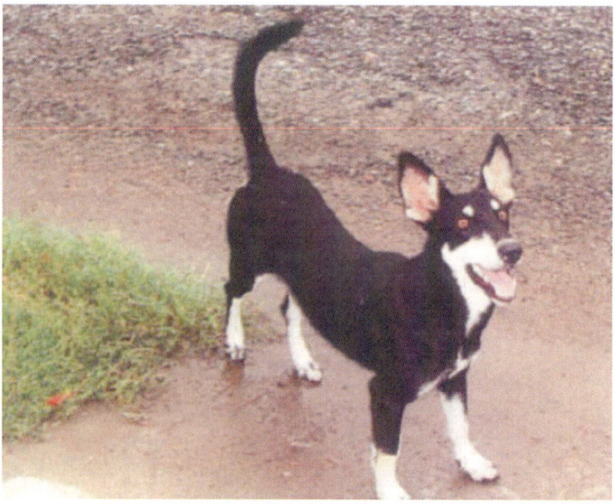

Fig. 2.49 Miniature Pinscher

12. **Pekingese :** According to a Chinese folk lore, this breed is a product of love a lion with monkey. It is a beautiful toy dog completely covered from top to botton in profusely growing long coat. Height is 15-25 cm and body weight less than 5.5 kg. Smaller size is preferred but in no case phenotype is accepted. All colours except liver and albino are accepted. Black mask is characteristic and feathered tail is carried high. (Fig.2.50)

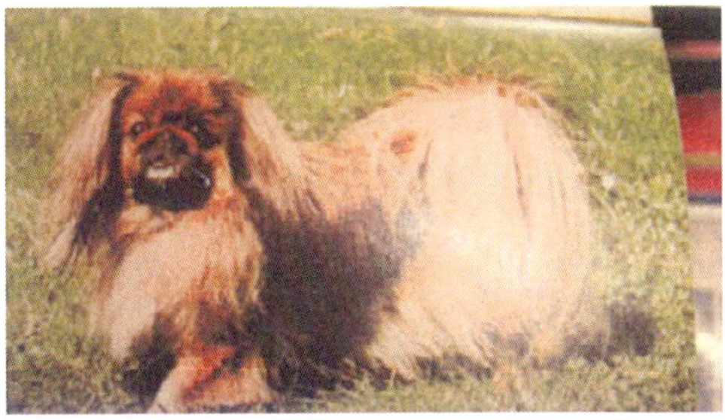

Fig. 2.50 a. Pekingese

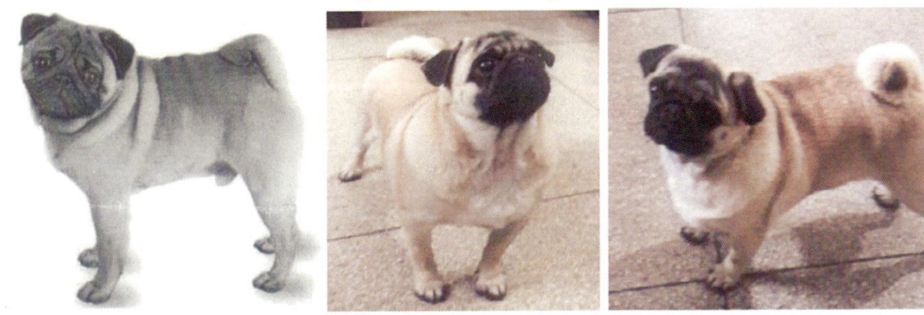

Fig. 2.50 b. Pug

13. **Pug:** This is a tiny bread of barrel shaped compact body and joker like blunt and black face. Skin is wrinkled at shoulders. Coas is short, dense and brown, limbs are strait and tail is coiled. (Fig. 2.50 b)

Few Indian Breeds

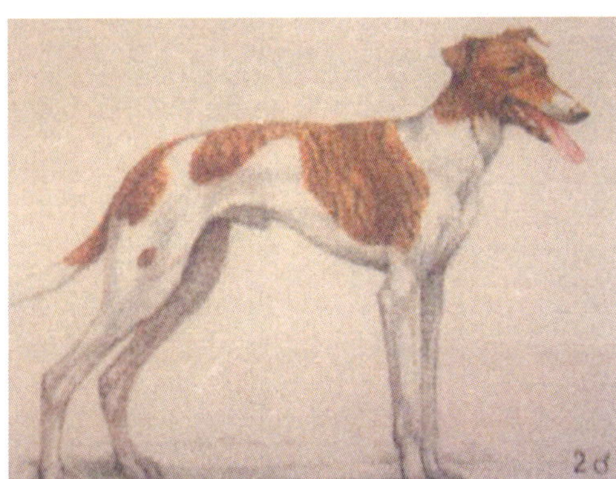

Fig. 2.51 Rampur Hound

1. **Rampur Hound:** It is a thin dog of light frame evolved by the Nawab of Rampur in Uttar Pradesh for assistance of hunting deer, antilope, etc. It is a slender dog of long limbs tucked up abdomen and stern tail. Body is coverd with short coat of variable colour.Whole colour animals are rare. Height range, 50-70 c.m. and body weight 25-35 kg. (Fig.2.51)

2. **Rajapalayam:** It is a hound of southern states specially the Tamil Nadu, Karnataka, and Kerala. The skull is domed and face is blunt. Body is long and compart with reasonably tucked up belly. Tail is long, tapering and upwards in the distal part. The dog was evolved for hunting wild games. (Fig. 2.52)

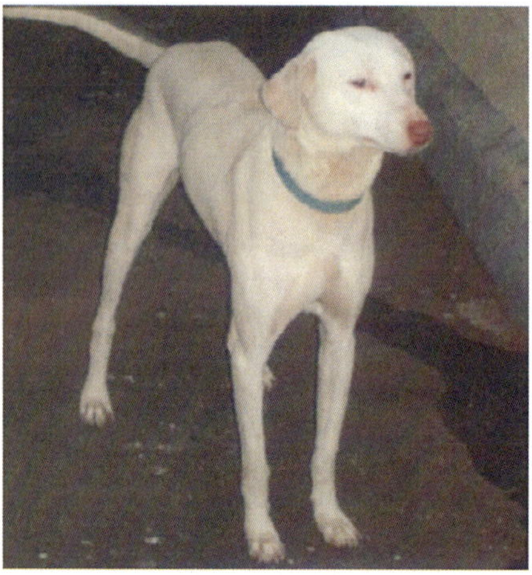

Fig. 2.52 Rajapalayam

3. **Mudhol:** The breed is popular in Karnataka and bordering Maharashtra and Andhra Pradesh. It is a popular watch dog or medium size. It was preferred for protecting the domestic livestock from wild and stray animals.The body is covered with short coat of black or tan colour.

4. **Gangetic Hound:** This breed is quite common along the basin of river Ganga and its tributaries. It is a medium size dog of black and tan colour, short body, coat round occiput and medium size dropped ears. The breed is more popular in rural areas and so far, it has not been described for fixing standard. (Fig.2.53)

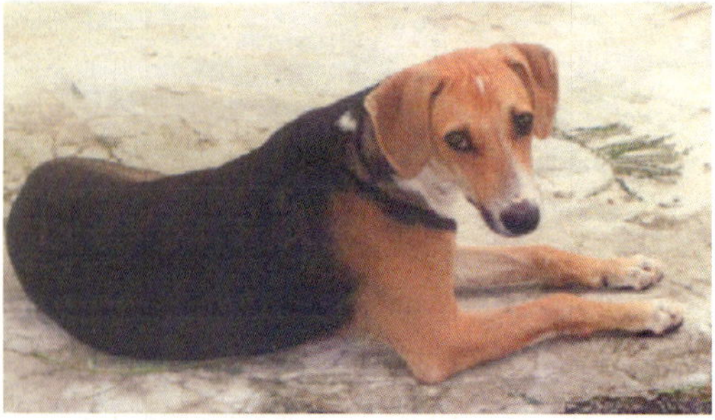

Fig. 2.53 Gangetic Hound

5. **Kombai :** It is a common house dog of Tamil Nadu famous for good nature and active habits. The faithfulness of dog has made it a good companion guard. Wedge shaped head and face is short, the eyes are bright and ears are common colour in different sheds of brown. (Fig.2.54)

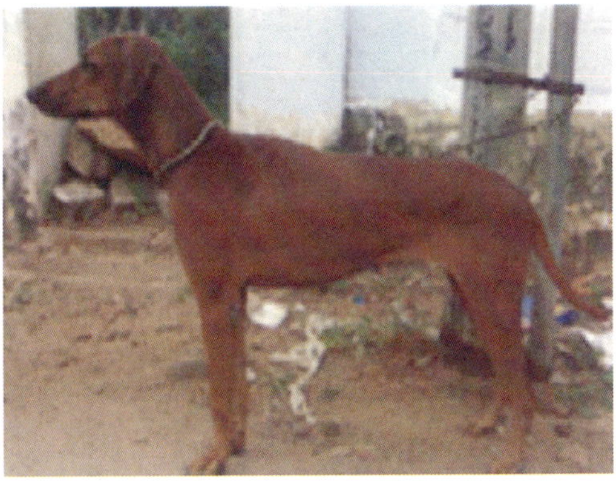

Fig. 2.54 Kombai

2.7 Brief Description of some Newer Breeds of Dog

Breeding of dogs for evolving newer synthetic breeds of dogs is a continuous process in developing countries. There are many newer breeds of dogs of Europe and America are less known in many countries. A brief description of some of the less known breeds is presented for information.

1. **Elo**: This is a new breed of Germany evolved by the Elo Breeding and Research Association. Its breeding was started during 1987 with main aim of developing a best pet fit for family environment. In the process of selection, more emphasis was given to nice behaviour than the phenotypic appearance of the dog. The size of breed is highly variable and in future, it may be differentiated into 2 or 3 strains or breeds. (Fig.2.55)

   Height of the breed: 35 cm to 60 cm

   Body weight: 10 kg to 35 kg
   Coat colour: It is a bicolour breed comprising of black and white, brown and white, grey and white, and red and white.

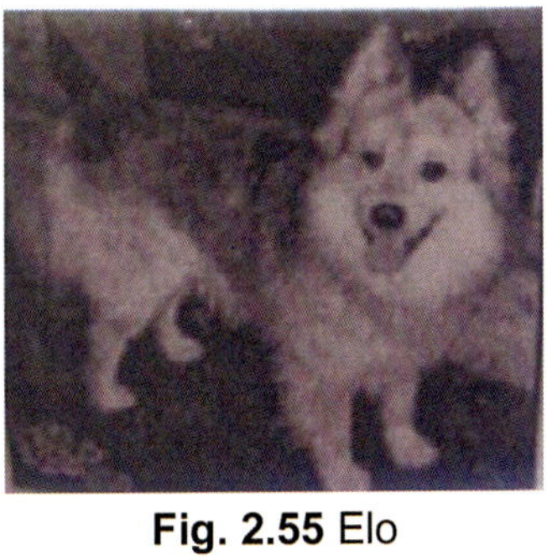

Fig. 2.55 Elo

2. **Thai Bangkaew Dog**: It is a medium sized spitz type breed of compact body of square shape.
3. **Turkish Shepherd Dogs**: These are 2 breeds (Kaugal Turkish and Akbash Turkish) following description:

Characteristics	Kaugal Turkish	Akbash Turkish
Birth weight (kg)	0.56	0.51
Weaning weight at 8 week (kg)	5.66	4.46
Body weight at 6 month (kg)	21.50	19.38
Body weight at 12 month (kg)	40.89	37.66
Height at shoulders (cm)	70.54	65.91
Height at rump (cm)	71.27	66.66
Body length (cm)	64.05	59.43
Circumference (cm)	78.10	71.86

4. **Shiloh Shepherd Breed:** The aim of breeding was to revive the traits of old German Shepherd breed as observed by Ms. Tina Barber in her childhood. It is a synthetic breed incorporating the traits of Old Wurttemberger, Malamute, a special cross breed of a Giant Malamute and an Alt Deutcher Shepherd in the German Shepherd.

   Shiloh Shepherd are available in 2 varieties, *viz:* (i) a smooth coat of medium length and (ii) a well-feathered coat. White coat colour is accepted only when nose, lips and eye rims are black.

5. **American Hairless Terrier:** This is the sole hairless breed of USA. It has been evolved from a mutant hairless female puppy born in 1972 in a litter of medium size Rat Terrier couple, which was back crossed with the father and produced only one hairless puppy in a litter of four. This was also a female. The bitch was then breed with her son and whelped one hairless puppy of either sex and two coated puppies. The breeding through selection was continued until establishment of traits.

   American Hairless Terrier is decorated with whiskers guard hairs on the muzzle and eyebrows. At birth, body is covered with sparse fussy hairs that start falling in a week after birth to complete by 6-8 weeks of age. The skin is very soft and smooth than the other hairless breeds. Ears are pricked and front facing. Tapering tail is carried high, if not docked. All types of skin colour are accepted.

6. **Dorset Old Time Bulldog:** It is a medium-sized dog with broad head, short muzzle, compact body, strong legs and smooth tail. The dog stands proud and fearless. The dog is strong, sporting and amiable.

7. **Tamaskan Dog**: It is a new wolf-like breed of lupine appearance without the addition of germplasm of a wolf. Tamaskan means 'mighty wolf' in the language of North American Indian. The dog appears like a wolf with dense and rough coat, small prick ears and blunt conical muzzle. The feathered tail is straight and should not be carried curled. Coat colour may be wolf grey, red or grey with black overlaying. Characteristic wolf like mask is a common feature. A faint ruff is present around the neck and shoulders to head. Profuse growing undercoat covers the body including inner surface of ears during the winter. Body length is more than the height. Almond shaped eyes may be yellow to brown. Blue eyes are disqualification. It is a good sledge dog, agile and obedient but not a good guard. The dog often turns unruly on longer rest period.

2.8 Some Synthetic Breeds of Domestic Dogs

The sources of germ plasm for the synthesis of dogs of desired traits are presented in the following table. Place of development has also be given for most of the breeds.

Table 1. Some synthetic breeds of domestic dogs

S.No.	Breed	Sources of germplasm	Place
1	Airedale Terrier	Old English Terrier, Otterhound and Welsh Terrier	Yorkshire
2.	American Water - Retriever	Irish Water Spaniel & Curly coated retriever	America
3.	Australian Terrier	Cairn Terrier, Dandies Dinmont Terrier and Maltese.	Australia
4.	Beagle	French Hound, Fox Hound & French Bulldog	England
5.	Black Terrier (Russian Terrier)	Two lines were used (i) Airedale Terrier and Giant Schnauzer and (ii) Giant- Schnauzer and Rottweiller	Russia

6.	Blood Hound	Ancient Celtic Hound & Mastiff	
7.	Boston Terrier	Bull Terrier, English Bulldog and French Bulldog	USA (Boston)
8.	Boxer	English Bulldog, Danziger Bullenbeiszer Brabanter Bullenbeiszer and Mastiff	Germany
9.	Bullmastiff	Bulldog and Mastiff	Europe
10.	Bull Terrier	English Bulldog and Terriers	UK
11.	Chesapeake Bay	Labrador, Irish Water Spaniel and Retriever Otterhound	USA
12.	Dobermann Pinscher	A stray dog crossed with Grey hound, Pointers, Manchester Terrier & Rottweiller	Germany
13.	Fila Brasiliera	Local Brazalian and Mastiff	Brazil
14.	French Bulldog	Small Mastiff, Griffon, Pug and Brabancon	France
15.	German Hunting Terrier	Smooth haired and Wire haired Fox Terrier, Welsh Terrier and Lakeland Terrier	Germany
16.	Gordon Setter	Collie, Blood Hound, Irish Setter and Pointer	Britain
17.	Great Dane	Mastiff and Irish Wolfhound	Germany
18.	Hungarian Vizsla	Yellow hunting dog, German Short haired Pointer, Hanoverian Schweisshund	Hungry
19.	Kerry Blue Terrier	Dark grey pups of Irish Terrier were breed with Bedlington Terrier, Dandy-Dinmont Terrier and Bull Terrier	England
20.	Labrador Retriever	Newfoundland and Pointers	England
21.	Leonberger	Landseer, Saint Bernard and Pyrenean Mountain Dog	Germany
22.	Pumi	Pomeranian and Briard	
23.	Shetland Sheepdog	Collie and Islanddk Hund or Yakki	Scotland

24.	Shih Tzu	Lhasa Apso and Pekingese	Tibet (China)
25.	Silky Terrier	Yorshsire Terrier, Skye Terrier, Scottish Terrier and Maltese	Australia (Sydney)
26.	Yorkshire Terrier	Skye Terrier, Dandies Dinmont Terrier and Maltese	Yorkshire

❑❑❑

Chapter 3

The Morphology of Dogs

3.1 Introduction

The wonderful world of dogs is quite fascinating, as despite similar anatomy and physiology, there is large variation in the shape and size of several hundred breeds of domesticated dogs distributed world wide. The size of domesticated dogs ranges from as little as rodent like tiny Mexican hairless dogs weighing few hundred grammes and the Chihuahua of about 1 kg to as large as 50 to 85 kg size of Mastiff, Leonberger, Great Dane and Saint Bernard breeds. Similarly, there is great variation in the height of dogs at shoulders and it ranges from as 15 cm in small Chihuahua to 90 cm in Great Dane. The variation in body coat colour is still higher which are solid or whole colour to shades and combinations of large number of colour. The size of coat ranges from hairless to short hair, medium hair, long hair, single coated and double coated breeds. Hairs of body coat are very fine, fine, silky, rough and coarse. The face may be blunt, blocky, wrinkles, smooth, broad, undershot or elongated narrow. The characteristics of shape, size, coat type, coat colour and markings have been either retained from the ancestors or have been significantly modified to the extent that in many breeds to the extent that it becomes often difficult to trace back the ancestors. The great changes in the shape, size, coat colour, coat size, texture of hairs, habits and behaviour of the domesticated dogs have been induced by the man through designed breeding programmes.

The modern domesticated dog of more than 400 breeds distributed through out the world are considered to be the descendents of different types of original native types of ancient wild dogs of Asia, Africa, Europe, America and Australia. For the development of newer breeds of desired traits inbreeding, cross breeding and rigorous selection have been extensively used for evolving the large number of modern breeds during the long period of 3 or 4 centuries in different countries. However, there are many stories about the utility of dogs during prehistoric era and mythology. The purposes of designed dog breeding had been highly variable from the development of fancy lap and tiny breeds to different breeds of utility dogs. During the development of new breeds and modified breeds, care has been taken to meet the requirements for adaptation with the various natural factors like climate, ecology, topography of location, the socio-cultural customs and the food habits of the human habitants of the locality. In the snow covered cold climate of the Siberian region heavily covered double coated breeds like Siberian husky, Eskimo and Samoyed, etc. have been evolved with soft, thick and dense woolly undercoat covered with outercoat of long and rough hairs for providing warmth and protection.

From the chilling cold breeze and snowfall through insulation. This protective trait is further intensified by the long outercoat that does not allow moisture to penetrate and wet the inner coat or body of the dog. The working breeds like Boxer, Great Dane, Collie, Alsatian, Mastiffs and Bhutia are mostly heavier with strong bonny and angulated limbs and also the indurance of walking long distance along with the herds and flocks on the grasslands and ranges. The hunting breeds like the Grey hound, Rampur hound, Saluki, Mudhol, Rajapalayam and Afghan hound are tall, narrow and slender animals with long and bonned forelimbs and well-angulated hind limbs suitably evolved for high speed and effective propulsion necessary for hunting. On the other hand beautiful breeds of tiny and small dogs are loyal, playful and obedient with pleasing disposition have been found to be excellent companion for all age group of people. The importance of this group has increased manifold in the urban areas due to working of most of the family members living behind the lonely elders and/or children in the home. The other factors for the popularity of small breeds are the isolated living, small family size, limited living space in the apartments and colonies, lack of time and field for the exercise of dogs, easiness of handling, less food requirement, ability to adapt the household food habits and good nature for providing company to lonely aged retired members and school going children in the family of most of the working couple.

3.2 Procedure of Description of a Domestic Dog

Detail description of different breeds and varieties of the dogs is required to be properly compiled for use at the time of identification and also for distinguishing the different breeds during the dog show.

After a series of exercise for hundreds of years now the widely accepted procedure for the description of a domesticated/pet dog has been standardized. The procedure is accepted by the kennel clubs as such or with little modifications to accommodate local requirements. Still sometimes minor descripancies surface due to some marginal differences in the shape and size accepted by the Kennel clubs of different places. The description of some of the recognized Indian breeds was started only during the nineteenth century, probably with the description of Rampur hound and the exercise is still incomplete due to which universely accepted description of the Indian breeds of dog is not available. This has adversely affected the reputation of Indian dogs and even the qualified veterinary graduates do not hesitate to write off the utility of Indian local dogs for efficiency, loyality, guarding, herding and retrieving, etc.

The morphology or phenotype and behavioural characteristics of a dog breed is described in such a manner to be useful in identifying the breed to a greater accuracy by a person not yet exposed to breed description. Normally, domesticated dogs are described in the following sequence:

1. **General characteristics:** These include informations regarding the origin, evolution, personality, behaviour, utility, popularity of the breed and sources of availability.

2. **Head (head and face combined):** The shape and size of head and face from the top of skull to point of the nose except the description of ears and eyes are included. There is great variation in the shape and size of head among the various classes and breeds of the dog.

3. **Mouth:** Mouth is usually included in the description of head but in some of the kennel clubs, it is described independent. It includes the description of jaws, lips, nose and arrangement of the visible teeth.

4. **Ears:** The description of ears includes the shape, size, disposition (erect or prick, half bent and hanging or drooping), placement on the skull and shape of the tip.

5. **Eyes:** The shape, size, placement and colour are normally included in the description of eyes. However, in some peculiar breeds and animals, the shape of orbit and eyebrows are also described.

6. **Neck:** The description of neck includes shape, size, arching, fusion with the shoulders and brisket alongwith coat type on the neck.
7. **Body:** The shape, appearance, arching, compactness and width from chest to waist, and finishing from withers to root of the tail are included in the description of body.
8. **Tail:** The description of tail includes shape, length, tapering, extent of curvature and coiling or curling, feathering, flag formation and placement, etc.
9. **Fore Quarters:** The description includes shape and sloping of the shoulders, compactness, boniness and size of the arms and fore legs, and flexibility of the pasterns.
10. **Hind quarters:** The shape and size of hips, thighs and hind legs alongwith their angulation are incorporated in the description of hind quarters.
11. **Feet:** The shape, size, arching and setting of toes, and padding of sole are included in the description of feet.
12. **Coat or Body coat (including colour):** The description of hairs covering the body includes length, lusture, texture and denseness.The coat may be single or double. In the double coated dogs, undercoat is soft, fine, dense and woolly. The colour of coat (outercoat in double coated) hair is either described alongwith coat or in some kennels separate. Markings on the body are also included in the coat colour.
13. **Shape and Size:** The height at withers and body weight are given in the description. The scales for measuring the height may be inches or centimeter and for body weight recording scale may be kilogramme (kg) or pound (lb). These values are given minimum, average or range, and may be separate values for either sex or the average of two sexes. The values are inter-converted, if needed and the figures are not rounded to next whole number-which are true transcription. This shows rigidity and marginal flexibility for rounding the values causing non-significant difference will be a more useful approach. For example, a height of 22.5 inches will be equal to 57.15 cm but it will be practical to use 57 cm. Likewise a 125 lb body weight is equal to 56.818 kg but it will be more practical to use 57 kg. Such minor descripancies due to inter conversion of units require to be rectified. In this book, recording has been rounded to 0.5 kg or 0.5 cm for all the dogs except the pups and tiny dogs below 5 kg body weight.

3.3 Description of a Dog (any sex) for Identification

Complete description of all official dogs employed in any service is maintained on an official proforma incorporating all aspects of physical characteristics of the dog. In addition to this, there are several occasions requiring the identification certificate of dogs from an authorized officer that is a registered veterinary practitioner. Some of the occasions requiring identification certificate are the registration, transportation, dog show, temporary housing in a dog hostel or admission in a nursing home as indoor patient. Earlier only few points like coat colour, eye colour and toes, etc. were recorded for identification but during the later half of the twentieth century, much elaborate method for the description of dogs has been evolved to facilitate easy identification in a group of dogs. The description of dog for identification may be preferably recorded in the following sequence or any suitable sequence specific for a state or country or registered kennel club:

1. **Name:** It should be routinely used name to which dog responds.
2. **Number:** In the dogs, numbers are not marked on the body surface and mostly collar tags are used. Moreover, it would be more useful to have a indeliable number by tattooing on under side of the tail near base or under side of the ear.
3. **Eyes:** The shape, placement and colour of the eyes are carefully recorded.
4. **Ears:** Like eyes the shape, size, placement and structure of ears are the main points to be recorded due to great variation between the breeds.
5. **Toe nails:** Colour of the nail of each toe is recorded.
6. **Breed:** It depicts the purity and recorded as pure, crossbreed or mongrel.
7. **Sex:** The dog may be male, castrated, female (potent bitch), spayed bitch or rig (single or double rig male). Rarely a dog may be hermaphrodite.
8. **Age:** Exact date of birth is recorded, when it is known. Otherwise it may be recorded as pup, young, yearling and adult dog or bitch on the basis of assessed approximate age.
9. **Coat:** The coat is first recorded as single coat or double coat and then the length of hairs (outer coat in double coated animals),

density, texture, fineness and others along with colour and markings are recorded.

10. **Markings:** These may be recorded separate, if not included with the coat colour. The hairs of different colour, shape and size than the basic coat colour are the markings. The markings may be beauty spot, star, stripe, blaze, mask, collar, saddle mark, blanket, kiss mark and shading, etc. The markings are acceptable in many breeds.
11. **Faults:** Any deviation from the standard in shape, size, coat, colour or any other characteristics of a breed is called fault. The faults are recorded for identification only and these are not accepted in standards breed. Such animals are not allowed to compete with the members of breed in a show.
12. **Faking:** The colour of coat, markings and toe nails should be examined carefully for attempts of masking or painting some accepted colour by dying. The shape of nails and ears may also be altered.
13. **Cosmatic changes:** Some kennel clubs have accepted defined cosmatic alterations in some of the breeds like characteristic hair dressing in poodles, docking of tail and cropping of earlobes.

3.4 Faking of Dogs

The intentionally induced alteration(s) in the morphology of a dog for hiding or removal of the non acceptable fault(s), changing some physical characteristics and altering some part of the body is known as faking. It is a malpractice and not acceptable for all purposes of competitive nature like dog show, etc.

Objective of faking: The main object of faking is to hide, mask, remove or rectify an unwanted phenotypic characteristic so that the animal is not debarred from the show. It is extensively used in pups for giving the appearance of a valuable breed for fetching higher price.

Methods of faking: The following methods are commonly used for faking the dogs:

1. **Use of physical methods:** The use of colour, cream and stiffeners is quite common for altering the colour of coat and texture of hairs.

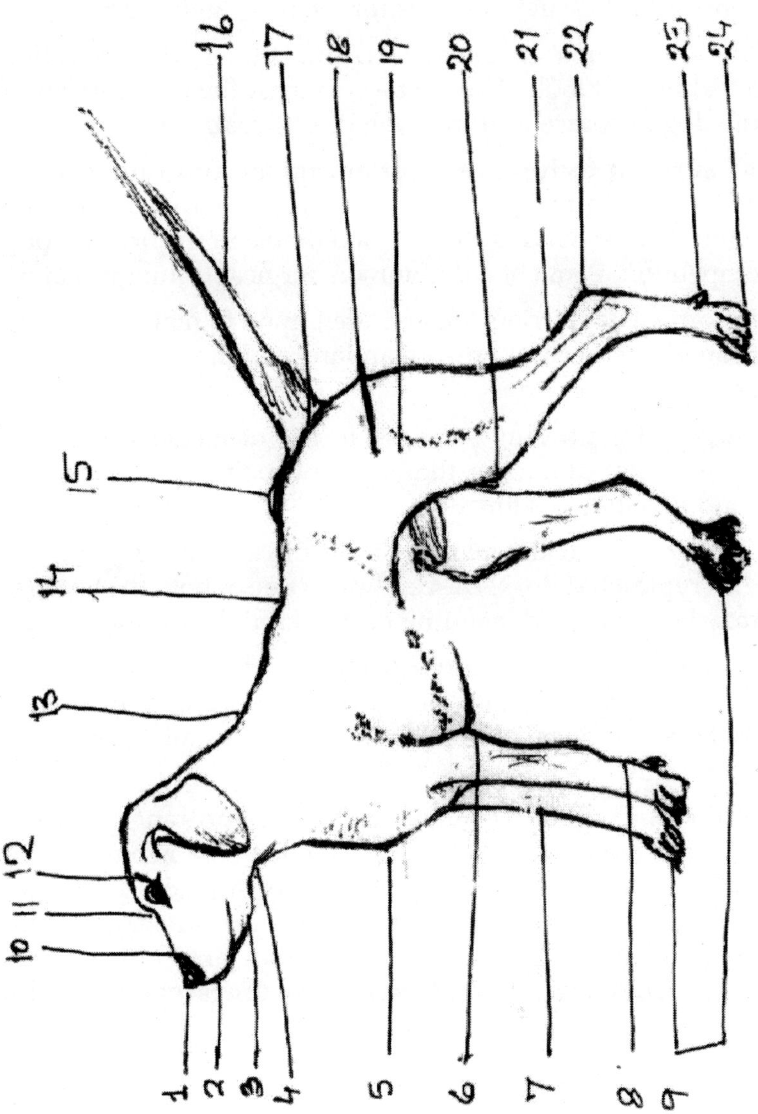

Figure 3.1 1. Nose 2. Upper jaw 3. Lower jaw 4. Throat 5. Chest 6. Elbow 7. Fore leg 8. Pastern 9. Toes 10. Muzzle 11. Stop 12. Eye 13. Shoulder 14. Black 15. Croup 16. Tail 17. Hip 18. Hip joint 19. Thigh 20. Stifle joint 21. Hind leg 22. Hock joint 23. Dewclaw 24. Paw

1.1 **Use of colouring agents:** Partial or complete dying of dog is practiced either for hiding or altering a disqualifying fault in coat colour or enhancing the physical look of the dog for attracting the attention of audience and the judges at the show. Extensive use of colouring is common in unregistered kennels and casual breeders for fetching higher price.

1.2 **Manipulation of coat texture:** Use of stiffeners for providing a feeling and look of coarseness to meet the requirement of the dog of coarse coat in a dog of soft coat.

2. **Use of surgical techniques:** Certain minor and rarely major surgical techniques are used for altering the undesired characteristics for making the dog acceptable in the breed group for competition. Some of the common surgical techniques are:

2.1 Deformed ear terriers are operated upon to make them fold properly as per the breed standard and also to keep them erect.

2.2 Surgery for proving strength to tail of terrier breeds for keeping standing over the back and pointing towards the head like that in squirrel.

2.3 To descend out the testicles from the abdominal cavity in the cryptorchid dogs. Descending of one or both the testicles may be required depending on the kind of cryptorchism.

2.4 **Correction of entropion or trichiasis in the eye:** Although this is a humane act for providing comfort to animal but it becomes faking on hiding. It is a hereditary fault transmitted genetically.

3. **Use of dooping agents:** The use of sedatives or tranquilizers in small dose is often practiced to hide the temperamental vice or undesired behaviour in a highly nervous or shy dog. The drugs are normally used during participation in show and transportation in a vehicle. Such dogs are not taken out at public gatherings. The marketing and use of these drugs for non-clinical purpose is a serious offence.

3.5 Terminology for the Stages of Life

Some of the common terminologies used for different stage of life and manipulations are given in Table 1. Many times some people use these terminologies also for cat. Therefore, for avoiding mingling terminologies for cats are also given.

Table 1. Common terms used for various stages of life cycle of dog and cat.

Stages and alterations	Dog	Cat
Any member of species	Dog	Cat
Intact male member	Dog	Tom
Breeding male	Stud dog	Tom
Female member	Bitch	Queen
Act of parturition	Whelping/Pupping	Queening
Offsprings/Newborns:		
a) Together	Litter	Litter
b) Individual of group	Pup or Puppy	Kitten
A group of animals	Pack	Clowder
Place of breeding/housing	Kennel	Home
Castrated male	Castrate	Neuter
Sterilized female	Spayed	Sterilized
Foetal membrane	Pup sac	Placenta
First milk	Colostrum	Colostrum
First faecal droppings	Muconium	Muconium
To stop suckling	Weaning	Weaning
Vocalization	Barking	Mew or Meo

3.6 Terminologies for the Body Shape of Dogs

1. Brachycephalic dogs = Synonym of Leonine dogs.
2. Brevilinear dogs = The body is much longer than the height.
3. Cloddy dogs = These are low set, broad or round and heavier dogs.
4. Cobby dogs = Breeds with compact muscular body, short back, deep chest and well spring ribs.
5. Dead straw = A dull straw colour dog.
6. Dolichocephalic dog = The dogs with narrow and long heads.
7. Elliptometric dog = The tiny breeds of dog.
8. Eumetric dogs = The medium sized breeds of dog.
9. Hypermetric dog = These are tall dogs.
10. Leonine dogs = The breeds with blunt, wrinkled and almost aquare head and very short face.

11. Mediolinear dogs = The breeds with narrow and long face.
12. Racy dogs = The tall breeds of light built.
13. Rangy dogs = The tall, long and slender breeds of dog.
14. Roach back dogs = The dog breeds with convex arched back.
15. Shelly dogs = A shallow and narrow body with too much tucked up and usually with insufficient amount of bones.
16. Slab sided dogs = The breeds with narrow chest due to less sprung ribs.
17. Spitz dogs = The breeds with almost square body.
18. Standard dogs = A dog as per official measurements for the breed, as prescribed by a kennel club.
19. Toy dogs = The tiny breeds of dog.
20. Tucked up body = A dog with pulled loin or lack of depth at the loin.
21. Wheet back = A strongly arched back like that of hyena.

3.7 Motion and Gait of Dogs

The movements and gaits of dogs are very important characteristics. These are given high emphasis during selection and training of the dogs. Special care is taken for the refinement of a particular gait in the working dog breeds. This also depends on the task to be performed by the dog.

Motion : The action of movement by changing the place or position is known as motion.

Locomotion : The act of movement from one place to another place with the use of own legs is called locomotion. It may be forward, backward or even sidewards. A forward progressive movement is a normal locomotion for a living creature like dog and others.

Movement: The entire process of changing of position from one position to complete in another position is known as movement. It is one of the important sign of life in a living subject.

Voluntary movement: The movement as per will of the subject is called voluntary movement.

Involuntary movement: Any movement of the body independent of the will of the subject is known as involuntary movement.

Gait: It denotes the co-ordination of stepping and movement. There are several types of normal and abnormal gaits in the dogs.

Gait or Gaited: These suffix are used to denote a gait,e.g., staggering gait, slow gaited and oxen gaited, etc.

Balanced gait movement:A balanced gait with perfect synchronization between the two halves of the body irrespective of the sides, whether the bisection is longitudinal or transverse, is known as balanced gait.

Non-slip retriever: The dog that stays at heels, marks the fall of game and retrieves to command.

3.8 Types of Gait

The gaits may be normal or abnormal. The normal gait is characteristic for the breed and abnormal gait are the deviations in normal gait. The causes of abnormal gait may be hereditary, congenital or acquired disorders in the dogs.

Types of Normal Gait: The terminologies used for the different gaits of horses are also used for the dogs with some alternate terminologies at some places as follows:

1. **Walk or Leisure gait**: The normal routine movement in the yard or outdoor. In this type of gait, the dog stops frequently at different places for knowing the immediate surroundings. They also urinate frequently, preferably on the prominent structures along the roads, streets or lanes etc. This is perhaps the marking of territory and also for remembering the route for safe return to home.
2. **Fast walk or Trot**: A moderate increase in steps per unit of time during the walk is known as fast walk or trot. The increase in steps should be 3 to 4 times depending on the requirements of trotting.
3. **The lope or Canter**: It is much faster than the trot and it is actually a kind of slow race.
4. **Fast run or Gallop**: The dog run to their maximum speed using all the four legs at a time.
5. **Single foot run** : Although this term has been used for high race but definition is not available. It may be superlative degree for gallop, in which all the four feet are lifted at a time from the ground.

Types of Abnormal Gait: Several kinds of deviation from the normal gait is seen in the dogs. These abnormal gaits are due to different kinds of hereditary, congenital, nutritional and acquired factors. Some of the common abnormal gaits are given as follows:

1. **Ataxic gait**: In this type of gait, the foot is raised high followed by the sole striking the ground at once and suddenly.
2. **Cerebellar gait:** There is lack of coordination in stepping while walking as observed in the case of alcohol overdosing or drunkenness. The main cause of such gait is different kinds of cerebellar disorders.
3. **Clipping gait**
4. **Crossing over gait:** To place one foot in front of another with a twisting motion. It is also called plaiting.
5. **Hackney gait (Action)**: Abnormal lifting of forelegs like a hackney pony.
6. **Heavy gait:** The dog moves reluctantly, as if the legs are packed with clay mud.
7. **Plaiting gait:** Synonym of crossing over gait.
8. **Slow gait**: It is an uncommon term sometimes used for lazy dogs.
9. **Spastic gait:** A movement in stiff manner with legs held closer or together. The toes seem to drag and catch.
10. **Staggering gait:** Synonym for ataxic gait.
11. **Stepage gait**: In this type of movement, the toes are lifted strongly and the heel reaches the ground first.
12. **Stilted gait:** The gait of a straight hock dog.
13. **Tabelic gait**: Synonym for ataxic gait.
14. **Waddling gait**: A duck like walking in the dogs suffering from pseudohypertrophic paralysis.
15. **Weaving gait:** Crossing the forefeet or hind feet while in motion.

3.9 Types of the Face

1. Blazed face = A large white patch on the face covering entire or large area of muzzle from the eyes to nose.

2. Blunt face = The oral end is broad, face bones are short and lips are generally thick.
3. Cheeky face = The bulging heavy cheeks as seen in obese dogs.
4. Chiselled face = A clean and smooth appearance of face down the stop.
5. Chops = Jowl and also the pendulous flesh of lips and jowl.
6. Cushion lips = Thickened upper lip as in Boxer, Pekingese and some others.
7. Dish face = A shallow concave forehead extending down to nasal bone.
8. Down face = Downward cuevering of nasal bone from stop to tip of the nose.
9. Elongated face = Narrow and long muzzle.
10. Elongated oval face = Stop is almost absent and oral end is rounded like an egg, as seen in Bedlington breed.
11. Fall = Long hairs falling on the face (hair lock).
12. Flare = A blaze wider at the top of the skull than between the eyes.
13. Frog face = An overshot upper jaw and extended nose.
14. Furrow = A streak (usually shallow) running down from occiput to stop.
15. Heavy face = The face bones are broad and covered with thick muscular layer.
16. Narrow face = Elongated face bones depict narrow and bony appearance.
17. Round face = The skull is large and the jaws are short and broad.
18. Thin face = Synonym for narrow face.
19. Throaty face or Throatiness = Loose heavy jowl, as in obese dogs.

3.10 Types of Head and Related Terminologies

1. Apple head = Domed or convex skull characteristic for some breeds but it is also congenital demormity in other breeds.
2. Brachycephalus = Broad and almost square head. Dog is called brachycephalic.

3. Crown = Top of skull between the base of ears. Synonym for occiput.
4. Dolichocephalus = Long head. Dog is called dolichocephalic.
5. Furrow = A depression line running down from center of occiput to stop.
6. Lean head = Head with little flesh and tight skin, as in Saluki.
7. Leonine head = Lion like head, as in Simhzhu breed.
8. Molera or Mollera = Deformed ossification of skull.
9. Occiput = Synonym for top or crown.
10. Peak = Synonym for crown or top or occiput.

3.11 Types of Eyes

1. Almond eyes = The upper curvature is more obtuse.
2. China eyes = Clear and small size blue eyes.
3. Ectopion = Outwards directed eyes.
4. Entropion = Inwards directed eyes.
5. Glass eyes = Wall eyes.
6. Haw = Nictitating membrane.
7. Orbit = Bony cavity on skull for housing eye.
8. Over hang = Prominent eye brow looming over a pushed in face.
9. Pearl eye = Glass eye or wall eye.
10. Pig eyes = Abnormally small eyes.
11. Super ciliary arches = Frontal bone of the skull forming the eye-brows.
12. Varminty = White or pale eye ball, may be complete, partial, unilateral or bilateral.
13. Wall eye = Synonym for glassy eye.

3.12 Terminologies for the Mouth Region

1. Bad mouth = Abnormal shape of mouth due to faulty denture. The shape is deviated from the typical shape of a breed.

2. Chops = Jowl. It is used for the pendulous flesh of lip and flew, as in Bull dog.
3. Deciduous teeth = Milk teeth or temporary teeth.
4. Even bite = Teeth of upper jaw and lower jaw oppose.
5. Eye teeth = Upper canine teeth.
6. Fangs = Canine teeth.
7. Flew = A pendulous lip of upper jaw overlapping the lower lip to different degree.
8. Hare lip = Cleft upper lip or even palate, as seen in hare and rabbit.
9. Hog mouth = The upper jaw is shorter than the lower jaw. It is also called undershot.
10. Incisors = Front row of teeth on jaws before the canine teeth.
11. Jaws = The bones of mouth holding the teeth.
12. Level bite = Synonym for even bite.
13. Lips = The free margins of oral opening made of epitheliomuscular tissues.
14. Lippy = A dog with pendulous lip.
15. Milk teeth = Deciduous or temporary teeth.
16. Muzzle = The lower part of face down the stop and forming the mouth.
17. Overshot = The upper jaw is longer than the lower jaw. It is also known as parrot mouth.
18. Parrot mouth = Synonym for overshot mouth.
19. Pig jaw = Similar to hog mouth.
20. Pincer bite = Synonym for even bite.
21. Scissors bite = The buccal side of lower incisors is covered by oral side or lingual side of the upper incisors.
22. Serrated lip = The margin of lip is serrated like a sickle.
23. Undershot = Synonym for parrot mouth.
24. Zygoma = Teeth bearing action of dogs.

3.13 Types of Nose

1. Butterfly nose = Partially pigmented nose like a black nose with pink area or pink patch.
2. Cherry nose = An off colour pink nose. It is disqualification for the Fox Terrier breed in many countries.
3. Duddley (Dudley) nose = Light brown or flesh colour nose.
4. Liver nose = A dull pinkish brown colour nose like that of liver.
5. Nose = The olfactory organ. Ability of a dog in identifying scent. On the basis of sensitivity, it is differentiated as:
   i) Great nose = highly sensitive scent differentiation power.
   ii) Poor nose = less sensitive power of scent differentiation, and
   iii) No nose = lack of scent differentiation ability.
6. Pink nose = Glossy pink colour of nose.
7. Roman nose = A convex and long nose bridge.

3.14 Types of Ears (Pinnae) and Ear Related Terminologies

1. Bat ears = Ears with broad base, rounded tip and short length with forward turned exposed ear canal.
2. Burr = Frontal aspect or inner surface of ear.
3. Button ears = Tightly folded compact ears placed on the skull like big buttons and pointed towards the eyes.
4. Drop ears = Pendulous or hanging ears.
5. Ears = For describing pina is called ear.
6. Ear cropping = Cutting ears to give specific shape or to make prick ear.
7. Erect ears = Pricked ears.
8. Flying ears = Folded or semi-folded ears, when stand erect.
9. Leathers = Long hanging or pendulous ears, as in Basset hound.
10. Prick ears = Erect ears as in Pomerenian, German Shepherd, etc.
11. Rose ear = A twisted or folded ear exposing the under surface.
12. Rounding of ears = Trimming of ear flap for making rounded shape.

13. Triangular ears = Ears with broad base and pointed tips.
14. Tulip ears = Slightly forward and curved cup-shaped ears.

3.15 Terminologies for the Legs

1. Angled = The bends at joints of hind legs.
2. Angulation = Same as angled.
3. Bandy legs = Abnormal outwards bending of one or more legs.
4. Barrel hocks = Outward turning of hock joints. It is also called spread hocks.
5. Bone or Boned = Well-calcified strong limb bones.
6. Cow hocked = A deformity of hind legs showing inwards bending of hock joints and outwards deflection of feet.
7. Crossing over = To place one foot infront of another with a twisting motion. It is also called plaiting.
8. Down in pasterns = Bending of fore legs due to the weakness or deformity of metacarpus bones.
9. Dysplasia = Loose set hip joint. It is mostly a congenital anamaly.
10. Fiddle = The feet turned inwards and elbows turned outwards.
11. French front = Fiddle front.
12. Gun barrel front = Straight fore legs. Synonym is plumb.
13. Hocks = The joint formed by distal extremity of tibia bone and proximal extremity of radius-ulna bones.
14. Huckle bones = The top of hip bones.
15. Lay back = The angle at which the shoulder blade (scapula) departs from the normal perpendicular position.
16. Leg = The organ of locomotion formed of a pair of fore or front legs and a pair of hind or rear legs.
17. Limb = Synonym of leg.
18. Loaded shoulder = Abnormally heavy shoulders.
19. Out of elbow = The elbow turning out of the body.
20. Pasterns = The joints made of metacarpus bones in front legs and metatarsus bones in hind legs.

21. Plaiting = Synonym of crossing over.
22. Plumb = The perfect vertical fore legs, also known as gun barrel legs.
23. Sickle hocks = Well let down hocks with strong angulation of both stifle and hock joints.
24. Splay foot = Flat foot with spread toes and paper pad.
25. Spread hocks = Synonym of barrel hocks.
26. Spread legs = Arched fore legs, as in Bulldog breed.
27. Stifle = The joint formed of distal extremity of femur and proximal extremity of tibia bone.
28. Straight hocks = Insufficient angulation of hind legs.
29. Terrier front = Straight profile at the front.
30. Timber bone = Leg bone.
31. Weaving = Crossing the fore feet or hind feet while in motion.
32. Withers = The dorsal border of shoulders.

3.16 Types of Tail and Related Terminologies

1. Bob tail = Natural born tailless puppy (freak) or close docked dog.
2. Brush = A bushy tail like that of a fox tail.
3. Coiled tail = A twisted curled tail formed of more than two tight curled rings.
4. Crank tail = A hanging tail.
5. Curled tail = A tail formed of 1, 3 or more rings.
6. Dock = Amputed tail stump.
7. Docking = Specialized (cosmatic or clinical) amputation of tail.
8. Dropping tail = Synonym for crank tail.
9. Feathering = Long hair cover on tail and other parts like thigh, legs and ears, etc.
10. Flag = Feathering of ventral aspect of tail. The longer hairs starting from the root of tail and gradually reducing towards the tip of tail.

11. Fringe = Feathering.
12. Gay tail = A tail carried curled over the back.
13. Kink tail = A short twist or bend in the tail.
14. Otter tail = A tail thick at the root and hairs parted on the under surface but not flagged.
15. Plumes = Soft and long hairs on the tail, as in bushy tail.
16. Pompon = Circular tuft of hairs at the end of the tail.
17. Rag tail = A tail with hairlrss tip
18. Rat tail = A tail with thicker root covered with curls and bare tip.
19. Ring stern = Curled or ring tail.
20. Ring tail = A curled tail carried over the back.
21. Sabre tail = Almost half-curled tail.
22. Screw tail = A short and screw like twisted tail.
23. Sickle tail = A semi-circular to inverted J-shaped tail.
24. Squirrel tail = A tail carried upright and then tilting over the back.
25. Stern = Whip like tail of a hunting breed.
26. Sting = A tail tapering to a fine point.
27. Tail = The organ made of coccigeal vertebrae.
28. Whip tail = Synonym of stern tail.

3.17 Terminologies for Body Coat and Hairs (Colour, Shape and Size, etc.)

1. Apricosa = Brownish orange coat (Apricot).
2. Apricot = Synonym for apricosa.
3. Apron = A frill of different colour on the chest and collar in same dog and it may extend upto the neck.
4. Beard = A tuft of specialized longer hairs on the chin.
5. Beauty spot = A coloured spot on white blaze on the forehead between the ears, eyes or face on the frontal bone.

6. Belton = A dense flecking of coloured hairs on the white coat. It appears ticking in short haired dogs but blurred in long-haired dogs.
7. Blanket = A different solid colour coat over the back covering larger area than the saddle.
8. Blaze = A large white patch on face covering greater or entire muzzle from eyes to nose.
9. Bloom = New crop of glossy coat replacing the shaded old.
10. Blue belton = Blue flecking on a white coat.
11. Blue merle = Admixture of black and white or grey hairs, as in blue roan.
12. Blue roan = Same as blue merle.
13. Bracelets = Ring of hairs left during hair dressing on lower part of legs below the knee and hock joints.
14. Breeching = Tan hair coat on the medial aspect of thigh.
15. Brindle colour = A combination of light and dark colouration of body coat forming irregular stripes. These are generally on brown, wheatish, grey or tan background.
16. Broken coat = Spoiled coat.
17. Clipping = Cutting of coat hairs.
18. Coarse coat = Body coat of rough and irregular hairs.
19. Coarse hairs = Hard and rough hairs.
20. Coat or Body coat = Hair covering on the body.
21. Coat colour= Colour of the hairs on the body.
22. Collar = A ring of white hairs around the neck.
23. Cullote = Very long hairs on the posterior aspect of thighs.
24. Curly coat = Hairs of body coat are twisted. Synonym for wire hair.
25. Dappled = Mottled markings of different colours without any predominance.
26. Dead grass = A dull straw colour dog.
27. Double coat = Two layers of different hair coats in double coated breeds. Under coat is soft, woolly and fine while outer coat is long and coarse.

28. Dressing = Cosmatic hair clipping or hair cutting.
29. Fall = Long hairs falling on the forehead as lock.
30. Feathering = Long hairs or tufts of long hairs on the body specially on the legs, ears, thighs and tail.
31. Felted coat = Mat formation of coat due to lack of grooming.
32. Flag tail = Feathering of under surface of tail with longer hairs starting from the root with gradual decrease in length towards the tip.
33. Flare = A different blaze broader at the top of skull than between the eyes.
34. Flecked = Sheding of the coat, when lightly ticked with other colour.
35. Foul colour = A typical coat colour or markings.
36. Frill = Long feathering around the neck with shorter hairs at throat.
37. Fringe = Feathering.
38. Furnishing = Profuse long hairs on certain parts of the body specially the fore face.
39. Grizzle = Bluish grey colour.
40. Guard hairs = Long hairs of outer coat for concealing the under coat.
41. Hackles = Erected state of hairs on the neck and back in a threatened dog due to fright or uncertainity.
42. Harlequin = Patched or pied colouration of a white or black ground colour like the dress of buffoons.
43. Haesh coat = A stif coat. It may be wiry also.
44. Hound markings = White, tan or black patches on the body.
45. Isabella = Fawn colour or greyish tello colour.
46. Kiss marks = Tan spots on cheeks and eyebrows.
47. Lemon colour = Light yellow coat.
48. Mane = Long hairs along the crest of the neck.

49. Mantle = Dark shaded portion of the hairs on the back and sides similar to blanket.
50. Marbled = Mottled coat colour.
51. Mask = Face colour different than the body colour.
52. Merle = Body coat of blue and grey hair mixture with black streaks.
53. Mis marked = Deviation of coat colour from the standard coat colour of the breed.
54. Molting = Normal and mostly seasonal shading of hairs.
55. Muzzle band = White muzzle.
56. Orange coat = Reddish yellow coat.
57. Parti-colour = Coat made of patches of two or more colours.
58. Penciling = Blue line on tan colour toes.
59. Pictus = Painted body coat, as in African Wild Dog.
60. Pied or Piebald = Parti-colour.
61. Pile = Dense under coat.
62. Plumes = Long and soft hairs on the tail.
63. Points = Colour of hairs on the legs, face, ears and tail.
64. Pompon = A circular tuft of hairs made at the end of the tail during hair dressing in some breeds.
65. Roan colour = Uniformly mixed coat of white and coloured hairs. It may be blue roan (mixture of black and white) or red roan (mixture of red or tan and white).
66. Ruff = Frill around the neck.
67. Rufous = Reddish brown.
68. Sable = A bright black hair lacing on light colour coat.
69. Saddle mark = A black or solid colour marking on the back like a saddle but smaller than the blanket.
70. Sedge colour = Dead grass colour.
71. Self colour = A single colour coat except for the shading.
72. Self marked = White or pale mark on chest, feet and either tip or under surface of tail on a single colour coat.

73. Shedding = Molting.
74. Single colour = Coat of any one colour.
75. Smooth coat = Uniform, short and dense haircoat.
76. Solid colour = Single colour.
77. Spectacles = Dark marking or shading around the eyes.
78. Splashed = Patches of white colour on solid colour.
79. Stand off coat = Long coat standing out from the body.
80. Staring coat = Bad or poor coat.
81. Stripping = Pulling out excess and unwanted hairs for thinning and smoothing the coat.
82. Texture if coat = Quality of coat hairs.
83. Thumb marks = Black marks on the pasterns.
84. Ticked coat = Small and distinct black or coloured marks on a white body coat.
85. Top knot = A tuft of long hairs made in the shape of a decorated knot on the top of head in some breeds.
86. Trace = Dark strip along the back. It is characteristic for pug.
87. Tri-colour = Coat hairs of three colours.
88. Trimming = Stripping or cutting the unwanted hairs of coat.
89. Under coat = Lower coat beneath the outercoat in double coated dogs.
90. Wheaten = Fawn or pale yellow tending towards red colour coat.
91. Whiskers = The neat and tidy beard of some terrier breeds. It is much less dense than the full beard.
92. Wire haired = Body coat of twisted hairs which are mostly rough.

3.18 Hunters Terminologies

1. Beagle = Small sized hound breed kept for hunting hares.
2. Cursorial hunter = Hunting by running.

3. Crop = A whip carried by the hunters.
4. Earth = Burrows of fox.
5. Form = Resting place of hare.
6. Harrier = A small fox hound used for hunting hares and rabbits.
7. Hunting crop = Hunting whip.
8. Pad = Foot of fox.
9. Sapling = A young grey hound.
10. Stopping earth = Filling in the earth for stopping a fox to enter its earth.

□□□

Chapter 4

Reproductive System of Dog and Reproduction

Basic informations about the reproductive systems of stud dog (male) and bitch are presented alongwith important aspects of reproduction.

4.1 Reproductive System of Stud Dog

The genital organs forming the complex tubulo-musculo-glandular reproductive system of stud dog are the operational parts and the accessory glands. The operational parts include the scortum, testicles and penis supported with ductus deferens, spermatic cords, urethra and prepuce. The accessory organs include prostate gland and uterus masculinus.

i) The Scrotum and Testes

The thin and soft skined smooth scrotum houses a pair of testicles. It is partitioned by a median septum into two sacs to hold testicle alongwith the epididymis and distal part of the spermstic cord in each sac. The scrotal skin is pigmented and oily on touch and posseses few scattered fine hairs on the surface and well-formed sebaceous and tubular glands.The scrotal raphe is generally faint in most of the breeds. The scrotum is placed posteriorly below the anus in the inguinal region. It is present in the shape of a tight projection in winter season due to contraction of the tunica dortos.

The testes descends in a pair of double-walled peritoneal sac known as processus vaginalis. The testes alongwith vaginal process are covered with abdominal fasciae which extend to cover the spermatic cords. A dortos is formed of smooth muscle fibres and collagenous and elastic fibres on the internal surface of scrotal skin. Internal abdominal oblique muscle extends posteriorly to form the cremaster muscle of the scrotum and fuses with the parietal vaginal tunic of the testes. The glandular skin with few scattered fine hairs, but without subcutaneous adipose tissue, alongwith contractile action of dartos and cremaster muscle the scrotum keeps the testes cool and functional. The scortum also provides protection from climatic factors, external trauma and other injurious factors to testes and associated organs enveloped in the sac. The blood is supplied by branches of external pudendal and femoral arteries and collected by the branches of testicular vein. Several fine branches of lumbo-sacral plexus (3rd and 4th lumbar and first three sacral nerves) innervate the different parts and organs of the genital system.

ii) The Ductus deferens or Vas deferens

The ductus deferens of each side is the exyension from the tail of the epididymis which is passage for the transportation of spermatozoa. The size of ductus deferens is highly variable and may be 16 to 20 cm long and 1.5 to 2.0 cm in diameter in the dogs of 10-15 kg body weight. These two ductus deferens converge about 2 cm prior to their opening into the prostate gland. These ductus are formed of tunica mucosa, tunica muscularis and tunica adventia from lumen to outer wall. The mucosal wall is formed of simple or pseudostratified columnar epithelium. The branches of prostate artery which is a visceral branch of internal iliac artery supplying blood, which is collected by the branches of spermatic vein. The branches of hypogastric nerve innervate the pelvic part of vas deferens while parasympathetic fibres join the epididymis and vas deferens.

iii) The Spermatic cord

These are two in number and each one is formed of vas deferens, testicular blood vessels and related nerve fibres enclosed in a cover of serous membrane. The spermatic cords start in the abdominal region and emerge through the deep inguinal ring to live the abdominal cavity at the distal end of ductus deferens. The various parts of spermatic cord join together by tunica vaginalis, which is made of loose connective tissue and peritoneum.

iv) The Prostate gland

It is only accessort gland present in the dogs. The prostate is a yellowish compact gland formed of muscular glandular tissue and enclosed in propimal part of the urethra. Near the neck of the urinary bladder. The prostate contains several buds of the pelvic urethra and its average weight is about 0.7 g per kg body weight of potent dogs in most of the breeds. A median groove shows the presence of two partition.

v) The Testicles (Testes)

These are two in number housed in respective scrotal sac. The shape of a testes is round oval and dorsoventrally thick. The size varies due to variation in body size of different breeds and much smaller in proportion to body weight. The testes are placed obliquely just below the anus. The length of testis ranges from 1.8 to 4.5 cm, width 1.2 to 2.8 cm and thickness 1.0 to 2.5 cm. Average weight of cleaned testes is 5.5 to 12 g. The testes are covered with tunica vaginalis and tunica albuginea. The testicular mass is made of numerous semi-niferous tubules glandular (Leydig) cells.

The three compartments of testes performing different functions are: (i) the basal, (ii) interstitial and (iii) adluminal. The functions of these compartments are controlled as well as feed-back by the two important glands, (a) the hypothalamus and (b) the pituitary (hypophysis cerebri) glands present in the brain. The Leydig cells are present in the interstitial compartment and synthesize testosterone, oestradiol and other hormones. The Leydig cells are also activated by the leutinizing hormone (LH) for the synthesis of pregnenolone from cholesterol and further metabolism of pregnenolone in the Leydig cells produces testosterone and oestradiol. The testosterone plays the main role of male reproduction. It is responsible for the growth of vas deferens and epididymis, initiation and maintenance of spermatogenesis and libido. The testosterone also regulates the secretion of gonadotropins releasing hormone (GnRH) by the hypothalamus and leutinising hormone (LH) and follicle stimulating hormone (FSH) by the hypophysis ceribri. The testosterone also regulates the growth of prostate gland and production of a prohormone for the synthesis of dihydrotestosterone and oestradiol. These two hormones are produced in the testes and peripheral tissues. These hormones act on the prostate gland for its maturation. Simultaneously, the growth of external genital organs is stimulated alongwith the appearance of secondary sex characters showing the attainment of puberty. Larger proportion of oestradio is synthesized from circulating testosterone by the process of aromatization and a small portion is produced by the testes in adult dogs.

The basal compartment is the second important functional part of the testes. It is formed of spermatogonia and Sertoli cells. From the lamina propria of the semi-niferous tubules of the basal compartment, cytoplasmic processes project from Sertoli cells in the lumen. The developing germ cells are placed on the basal and adluminal compartments of the testes. The functions of Sertoli cells is controlled by the action of FSH and testosterone. Various substances required for the spermatogenesis are synthesized by the Sertoli cells, which are also necessary for the maturation of spermatoids. The FSH acts on the Sertoli cells which consequently stimulates the germ cell and its specific function depends on the growth stage of germ cell in contact with the Sertoli cells.

The oestradiol produced by Leydig cells is transformed into testosterone by the action of the Sertoli cells, which is more consipicuous in the pre-pubertal growth. Greater proportion of testiculae oestradiol in adult dogs appears to be produced by the Leydig cells. The functions of oestradiol in the reproduction processes of male dogs are not yet clearly known. However, in conjuction with testosterone, it is involved in the regulation of secretion of the gonadotropins. In the prostate gland, oestrogen increases the production of androgens by regulating the number of dihydro-testosterone receptors.

There is overlapping in the functions of second and third compartments. A special protein, androgen binding protein is also synthesized by the Sertoli cells which is responsible for moderating the action of testosterone. It is also considered to be associated with the transportation of testosterone within the testes and epididymis. The two hormones involved in the regulation of FSH secretion are also produced by the Sertoli cells. The activin hormone increases the secretion of FSH by the hypophysis cerebri (pituitary gland), whereas inhibin decreases. A Mullerian inhibiting biochemical is also produced in the Sertoli cells of foetii and young prepubertal dogs. This substance is responsible for the regeneration of the Mullerian ducts during the process of sexual differentiation in the embryos.

vi) The Urethra

It is a common passage for the routine excresion of urine and also the semen via a pair of ductus deferens at the distal end of the pars longa. The size of urethra may be 10 to 35 cm in different breeds. The three parts forming the urethra are the prostatic part, membranous part and penile part. There is an oval seminal hillock, colliculus seminalis in the centre of the urethral crest on which a small tube opens from the uterus masculinus and ductus deferens drains on either side of the hillock.

The blood is supplied by the branches of prostatic and urethral arteries and drained by the branches of veins from the prepuce.The urethra is covered by a small size bulbo-cavernosus muscle and the strong urethral muscle. The ischio-urethral muscle originates from the tuber ischii and inserts on a fibrous ring present at the symphtsis ischii. The dorsal vein of penis is enveloped by the muscular layer.

vii) The Penis

The penis of dog is different in structure than the organ of other mammalian species. Like other organs of dog, the size is highly variable. It may be 5 to 25 cm long in tiny toy breeds to heavy tall breeds. The penis can be differentiated into three parts, *viz.* the root, the body and the glans penis. The posterior part upto body is made of corpora cavernosa, corpus spongiosus, penile urethra and enlarged anterior part containing os penis. The os penis is considered as a ossified portion of the corpus cavernosum and its length may range from 2 to 10 cm in different breeds. The corpora cavernosa are distinguished by a median septum and innervated by many venous spaces. The corpus spongiosum present in a groove covers the penile urethra. The glans penis is longest of the three parts of the penis and can be differentiated by a bulbus glandis and the pars longa glandis. The posterior one third part of pars longa glandis covers the anterior half of the bulbus glandis. A connective tissue septum separating these two organs also forms a cover for the corpus spongiosus and the os penis. The bulbus glandis and pars longa glandis are formed of erectile tissue. The os penis is thicker dorso-ventrally, tapering distally, grooved ventrally for the placement of urethra and ends as a little vurved fibrocartilaginous projection. The glans penis is highly vascular. The os penis helps in intromission without erection, which occurs subsequently. The enlargement of bulbus glandis during the erection of penis does not allow the withdrawl of penis during semen ejaculation. At the time of copulation, the blood engorgement of cavernous space provides rigidity to penis.

viii) The Uterus masculinus

It is a tiny compact rudimentary remains of the paramesonephric duct present in the colliculus seminalis. It is formed on the dorsal aspect of the posterior part of the urinary bladder and anterior part of the prostate gland.

ix) The Prepuce

It is a complete tubular sheath that covers the penis. The inner part of prepuce is pinkish in colour and glandless. It is formed of a thin layer of stratified squamous epithelium. The outer layer of prepuce is an extension of the abdominal skin.

x) Puberty in male dogs

Under optimum feeding and management, puberty is attained at 9 to 12 months of age in different breeds. The process may be a little earlier in the pups reared in the group of mixed sexes.

4.2 Effect of age on Spermatogenesis and Sexual Behaviour of the Dogs

1. Initially, semen quality improves rapidly in early life following puberty and good quality is maintained upto 6 to 8 years in different breeds.
2. The stud dog remains very active and aggressive in young age. However, nature of shy dogs is generally avoiding and compromising with the aggressive one.
3. The semen production and fertility of dogs remain even in most of the aged ones but participation in active mating decreases.
4. Geriatric males are mostly found reluctant for mating even with the bitches in standing heat. The other factors in competitive street dogs are the appearance of more active and aggressive behaviour of younger dogs. Such potent dogs are preferred by majority of eligible bitches.

4.3 Mating Behaviour of Male Dog

The aggressive and dominant characters of a dog determines its scope of mating. Such dogs do not allow others for mating with the bitches of their territory, if they are not tied with a bitch. This is reflected by the birth of greater proportion of puppies exhibiting some of the phenotypic traints in a colony or locality having many street/ stray dogs and bitches. The traits transferred from sire to off springs may be colour, shape of face, ears, eyes, tail etc.

In the free living dogs the dominance is established and territory is marked where other dogs are not allowed trespassing. An outsider is immediately chase out by the dogs of locality. In each colony of street dogs there is a dominant male which is generally most robust, active and intelligent in the group. Most of the progeny is sired by such dogs. In kennels it is the prepotency of stud dogs that determines the phenotype of progeny. The choice of stud dog in kennel is decided by the owners of bitches. Sometimes owners seek the advise of master of the kennel.

4.4 Age of Stud Dogs for breeding and breaking of First timers

The stud dogs are introduced to mating only after 12 months of age and preferably after 14-15 months of age. The stud dog should grow to attain the standard shape and size of the breed before breaking for breeding. The stud dogs should be maintained in good health and should be frequently examined for sexual health also before the onset of breeding season. The first timer stud dog should preferably be introduced to a docile and experienced (in 2nd to 4th parity) bitch a few days before the standing heat. Unexposed young males, when allowed mating for the first time, they make several unsuccessful attempt to mount and hold the bitch for intromission. Only few succeeds on co-operation of bitches, whereas many exhaust in the attempt of first time mating. In case of kennel stud, this exposure should be short to avoid the frustation due to unsuccessful mating. An aggressive and young bitch should not be introduced to a first timer stud because many times delay in intromission infuriate aggressive bitches and they may injure (bite) the young stud. Such bitches often injure the testes.

It is advantageous to introduce the inexperience stud to bitch at the beginning of proestrous. The introductory meeting should be of short duration starting with 10-15 minutes on first day to maximum 30 minutes. These meetings provide opportunity for developing some friendly relationship to facilitate consummation on oestrous. Care should be taken to prevent fighting during the pre-copulation meetings because any attempt to copulate before the true oestrous is not acceptable to a normal bitch and stud may be injured by sudden biting.

4.5 Approach of Stud Dog for Mating

At initial meeting, the stud dog first approaches the face of bitch and if allowed, then licks and rubs the face. After this, he attempts for smelling and rubbing the perineal region. In case of street dogs, many males run behind a bitch right from the start of the proestrous and during the period dominance of a capable male is established but others continue to move in the group. During this period, many virgin and experienced bitches not yet in any stage of oestrous cycle do not attract any male.

4.6 Mating (copulation or coitus)

In the dogs and other canines, a bone os penis maintains the rigidity of penis, which helps in intromission of penis into the vagina before actual erection. During the process of erection, the bulbus glandis of the penis enlarges 2-3 folds due to engorgement of blood filling the vestibule. This prevents the seperation of copulating pair. The ejeculation of first two fractions of the seminal fluid starts immediately after the intromission of penis into the vagina by the very speedy thrusting. After this pelvic thrusting is ceased and male turns in opposite direction while dismounting and remains in this tail to tail position for quite some time. The faces of two partners are away but erect penis turns almost 100 degree in horizontal line. This is known as locking position or post coital lock or tie position. In locking position, ejeculation of the third fraction of seminal fluid (prostatic fluid) occurs. The tie position continues for sometimes which is normally 15 to 30 minutes but may be even longer in some cases. Tied pair of street dogs may be observed dragging, if disturbed by humans or other animals.

Intromission of penis is not completed in case of prior erection. In such cases, post coital locking does not occur. In casual terms, such situation is called outside tie. The mating male is unable to deposit total seminal ejeculate in the vagina of the bitch.

4.7 Semenology

In the dogs, semen is discharged in three fractions. The first smallest fraction of only few drops is considered to be secreted from the prostate gland. The quantity may be few mililiters in some of the dogs. This fraction is known as presperm fraction. This is followed in continuation by the second fraction, which is concentrated with spermatozoa. The volume of second fraction ranges from 0.5 ml to

5.0 ml or even more in some exceptional large dogs. The volume of second fraction depends on the size of testes, age of the dog and individuality of the dogs. This fraction is cloudy milky and opalescent in appearance. The two fractions are not separated during semen collection in the artificial vagina. The volume of third fraction is largest ranging from 5 to 30 ml and secreted by the prostate. This fraction is clear and different from the cloudy second fraction. This fraction is collected to ensure the collection of all spermatozoa of the ejeculate.

4.8 Purpose of Semen Collection

1. For use in artificial insemination.
2. For preservation and conservation to facilitate use for longer period or even after the death of a prized stud dog.
3. For the evaluation of fertility of a stud dog.
4. For the evaluation of semen quality.
5. For the diagnosis of ailments of the male genital organs.

4.9 Parameters of Semen Quality Evaluation

1. Volume of ejaculate in relation to breed. 10 (1-26) ml
2. Colour of the semen. White to creamy
3. pH: 6.7 (6.0-6.8)
4. Concentration of spermatozoa per ml of semen and per ejeculate. 125 (20-540)
5. Motility of spermatozoa: It should be more than +3 on 5 point scale or > 60%. But preferably > +4 or > 80%.
6. Morphology of the spermatozoa, *viz:*
   a) Percentage of normal and/or abnormal spermatozoa: Abnormal spermatozoa should be less than 10% in fresh ejaculates.

   b) Types of abnormalities of spermatozoa. These are headless, tailless, double head, coiled tail, elongated head, double tail, etc.

   c) Percentage of live and dead spermatozoa. In fresh ejaculate, live spermatozoa should be more than 70% and preferably more than 90%.

7. Semen cytology for the detection of cells other than the spermatozoa: Semen should be free from blood cells, pus cells and cell debris.
8. pH of fresh semen and diluted (extended) semen.
9. Alkaline phosphatase in semen.
10. Hormonal assessment of the semen for testosterone, luteinising hormone (LH) and follicle stimulating hormone (FSH).
11. Microbiological examination for the detection of: (a) normal flora and (b) the pathological flora.

4.10 Selection and Management of Stud Dog

Following criteria should be considered for the selection of stud dog:

1. The morphology must be breed specific and ancestory records should be available at least upto grand parents of dam and sire.
2. The dog should be more active and intelligent than the average of the breed.
3. The dog should be sound and free from genital abnor,alities like phimosis, paraphimosis, cryptorchidism (unilateral or bilateral).
4. The puppies are selected at young age of 3-4 months, so that rearing can be possible under standard feeding and management. Stud dogs are fed half cooked meat to constitute more than half of the daily ration during the growing period. The diets should be balanced for minerals and vitamins and should also contain sufficient dietary fibre for the normal passage of digesta and evacuation of bowel.
5. Adequate exercise should be provided daily and quantum should be optimum for the breed, *viz.* 30 minutes fast walk for small breeds, 45 minutes for medium breeds and 60 minutes for large breeds. Some hounds and working breeds require more rigorous exercise and laxity may cause obesity. The exercise may include running and playing also. The time of exercise should be morning and evening before feeding.
6. Optimum body condition should be maintained. A marginal lighter stud is generally more efficient breeder than the flabby obese dogs.

7. If an apparent healthy stud dog fails to produce progeny or fertilizes, only few of the covered bitches should be removed from the breeding group. Nutritional management and hormonal treatment may improve the breeding efficiency of such dogs.

4.11 The Female Dog (Bitches) Reproductive System and Reproduction

The reproductive system of bitch includes a pair of ovaries, a pair of oviduct (uterine tube or fallopian tube), the uterus including the two horns, the vagina, the vulva and associated structures of specialized tissues. The abdominal parts of the reproductive system are hold hanging from the abdominal ceiling by the broad ligament. The mammary glands are also considered alongwith the true reproductive organs because these are very important for nursing the puppies in early life.

i) The Broad Ligament

It is a paired double fold peritoneum that holds and attaches the reproductive organs with the ceiling and lateral walls of the abdominal and pelvic cavities. The three parts of broad ligament holding the ovaries, the oviducts and the uterus including the uterine continuation of vagina are known as mesovarium, mesosalpinx and mesometrium, respectively. The blood vessels and nerve branches of the reproductive organs are present embedded in the broad ligament.

ii) The Ovaries

These are two in number located in the abdominal cavity, somewhere in the area of third to fourth lumbar vertebrae near the posterior border of the either kidney. The ovaries are elongated bodies of variable size. The size varies due to great difference in the body size of bitches of different breeds.The average length, breadth and thickness of ovaries of an adult bitch of 10 to 15 kg body weight may be 1.3-1.7 cm, 0.6-0.8 cm and 0.4-0.6 cm, respectively. The average weight of each ovary ranges from 250 mg to 400 mg. The surface of quiescent ovaries of young pre-pubertal bitches are smooth, which become rough in sexually mature bitches due to development of follicles of different size and subsequent formation of spots of recession of corpora lutea in the breed bitches. The right ovary is situated between the right arm of the duodenum and the right lateral abdominal wall. The left ovary is present near the lateral aspect of the spleen. Each ovary is contained in peritoneal pouch called bursa overii and formed of two layers containing sufficient adipose tissue and unstratified muscle. A slit like opening is present on the ventral aspect of the pouch. The peritoneal pouches further extend to make mesosalpinx attaching the uterine horn and the ligaments of the ovaries. The ovaries are suspended by the meso-ovarian part of the broad ligament.

The functional parts of ovaries are constituted of two parts: (i) the cortex and (ii) the medulla. The cortex is formed of a connective tissue stroma. The medulla is supplied with arterial and venous blood vessels and the nerves which are continued in a core of connective tissue and muscle fibres. The basement membrane of the cortex contains large number of germinal cells, which develop into follicles after the onset of puberty. On the maturation of follicles, ovulation occurs and corpus luteum is formed from the wound made due to ovulation. In non-breed bitches, the corpus luteum regresses into a scar called corpus albicans but in breed bitches regression occurs only after whelping. The blood circulation is maintained by ovarian branches of the uterine artery, vein and the lymphatics open into the lymph nodes of lumbar region. Branches from the renal nerve and aortic nerve plexus innervate the ovaries.

iii) The Oviducts or Fallopian tubes

These are two in number and located on either side. The length ranges from 4.5 cm to 8.0 cm in different breeds. The oviduct is made of an infundibulum and a tortuous connective tube. The funnel shaped infundibulum is decorated with several motile fimbriae, which help the capture and transportation of ova into the uterine cornua through the oviduct by peristaltic movement. The fertilization mostly takes place in the uterus. The three types of tissues forming the outer, middle and luminal layers are the fibrous tunica serosa, the tunica muscularis of circular, longitudinal and oblique fibres of smooth muscle, and the tunica mucosa of partially ciliated simple columnar epithelial cells, respectively. The cilia of luminal mucosa move towards the uterine horn during ovulation. The blood supply is maintained by the branches of ovarian and uterine arteries and veins. The nerve fibres from the renal and aortic plexus innervate the ovaries.

iv) The Uterus

The uterus is made of three parts, *i.e.* the cervix (neck of uterus), the corpus uteri (body of uterus) and a pair of uerine cornua (uterine horns). The organ is more or less Y- shaped. The horns extend anteriorly to form the oviducts of respective side. The posterior end of corpus uteri forms the cervix opening into the vagina. As usual, the size of uterus is highly variable being small in smaller breeds and large in larger breeds. In a medium size adult bitch, the body of uterus is only 2-3 cm and non-gravid horns may be 10-15 cm long. The horns are uniform tubular structures situated in the abdominal cavity and two branches diverge towards the respective kidney. The cervix is very short and muscular, and projected slightly into the vagina. The volume of uterus increases with the increase in age, onset of puberty, number of parity and the stage of pregnancy (in pregnant bitches).

There are three openings in the corpus iteri, *i.e.* one each of uterine horns is called ostium uteri and third one is the ostium uteri externum opening through cervix into the vagina. The wall of uterus is made of three layers of different tissues, *viz.,* the outer fibrous tunica serosa, the middle thicker layer of tunica muscularis or myometrium and the luminal layer of tunica mucosa or endometrium. The endometrium is lined by a layer of ciliated low columnar epithelium. Several branched and coiled uterine glands present embedded beneath the tunica mucosa open on the luminal surface. The blood circulation is maintained by the ovarian and uterine blood vessels. The lymphatics open into the hypogastric and lumbar lymph glands. Fine branches from the hypogastric plexus and the pelvic nerves are distributed in the uterus.

v) The Vagina

A relatively long musculo-membranous tubular structure connecting the uterus at the cervix anteriorly and the vulva posteriorly is the vagina. It is the organ of coitus. The vagina is narrower towards the cervix uteri and does not possess well-defined fornix. A definite hymen is not present in the bitches. From exterior to luminal surface, the organ is covered with tunica serosa, tunica muscularis, tunica propria and tunica mucosa. The tunica mucosa is made of non-glandular stratified squamous epithelium. The luminal surface of the vagina forms several longitudinal folds. The blood circulation is maintained by the vaginal branches of internal pudendal artery and veins, and the lymphatics drain into internal iliac lymph glands. Many fine branches of nerves are supplied by the pelvic plexus and the pudendal nerve.

vi) The Vulva

The vulva is formed of vestibule, clitoris (the rudiment of male organ) and labiae. The vestibule is a small passage connecting the vagina with the vulva. The external urethral orifice opens on the urethral tubercle, a shallow ridge like projection on the ventral surface of the vestibule. The clitoris is a shallow button-shaped projection of highly sensitive tissue at the narrow end of the vestibule. The external rim of the vulva is formed of the vulvar labiae which join together to form dorsal and ventral commissures. The ventral commissure is projected downwards. The clitoris is present in fossa clitoridis at the terminal point of the vestibule. It is formed of a pair of crura clitoridis, corpus clitoridis and glans clitoridis. The body of clitoris is composed of mainly adipose tissue containing few fibres of erectile tissue and it is covered by a thick tunica albuginea. Presence of os clitoridis is very rare in few bitches and it does not interfere in normal coitus. The inner surface of vulva is made of stratified aquamous epithelium containing variable number of lymph glands. The intermediate muscular layer is the continuation of tunica muscularis of the vagina with some additional striated circular muscle, the constrictor vestibular muscle and the constrictor vulvar muscle. The ischio-urethral muscle originating from the posterior-medial surface of the tuber ischii are inserted in the less developed central tendon of the perineum. A small ischio-cavernosus muscle originates from the posterior border of the ischium and inserts at the crura clitoridis. The orifice of female urethra possesses a strong muscular sphinctor.

The blood is supplied by the branches of vaginal artery and the internal and external pudendal arteries. The return of venous blood is carried by the lateral veins into the pudendal vein. The lymph vessels open into the superficial inguinal lymph glands. Fine branches of the pudendal, genital, hypogastric and pelvic nerves extensively innervate the organ.

4.12 Puberty in Female Dogs (Bitches)

The age of bitches at puberty is highly variable due to great difference in size, longevity and management of the animals. It is generally earlier in street dogs, where female and male pups live and grow together in the group of adults. Some of the factors affecting the age at puberty are the breed, environment, plan of nutrition, climate and management. The onset of puberty is much earlier in small breeds and its duration normally increases with the size of breed. The age at puberty ranges from 6 to 12 months. In some heavy breeds, it may considerably extend beyond 12 months. The onset of puberty is normally earlier than the male littermate and same breed kept in common management.

4.13 The Oestrum or Heat in Bitches

1. A bitch comes in heat at an interval of 5 to 8 months after the onset of puberty.
2. The duration of oestrum is about 3 weeks.
3. A few bitches show heat only once in a year while few rare with infantalism never show oestrum. Such bitches need veterinary aid, if oestrum is not exhibited upto 14-15 months of age.
4. Signs of oestrum (heat) in bitches are:
   a) Swelling of the vulva with glossy appearance.
   b) Initially vaginal discharge is almost colourless. After few days, the vaginal discharge becomes pinkish red and later, it becomes blood stained. These changes occur due to erosion of the uterine wall in preparation for the attachment (implantation) of the fertilized eggs (now zygote) which will subsequently develop as foetii.
   c) The coloured discharge may continue upto the middle of the oestrus duration and then diminishes leaving again a colourless mucous which lasts until the end of the heat.
5. The bitch is usually ready to be breed, when colour of vaginal discharge begins to subside. This is normally from 7 day of heat to end or one day before the end of oestrus. Only a rare few may allow mating earlier or later, and this is not an abnormal behaviour.
6. Ovulation in bitches occurs, when mating is allowed. The mature ova are held in the fallopian tubes, where they remain until fertilized.
7. In a non-breed bitch, all ova degenerate and expelled out of the body as a waste.
8. A bitch in season (heat) must be carefully looked after and should not be given the opportunity to escape to find her own mate.

The pet bitch in house should be kept secured. An anti-male chemical may be sprayed around the tail region for repelling the male dogs.

9. A bitch in heat should not be allowed to contact chill by lying on cold or wet ground of concrete or marble or stone slab in a yard or kennel run.
10. The bitches in heat should be provided shelter for protection from cold wave in chilly winter season. Negligence may cause reproductive disorders like vaginitis, metritis, etc. Sometimes, it may be serious requiring hystrectomy.
11. In case of misalliance, an injection within 48hours of mating can be effective to stop pregnancy. The drugs (abortificients should not be used repeatedly.

4.14 The Oestrous Cycle

The bitches are seasonal breeder and oestrous cycle appears twice annually in most of the bitches. The interval between the successive oestrous cycle may be 5 to 8 months (average 7.5 months) in different breeds and under different management and climate. The oestrous cycle may start any time in a year but in the tropical plains of India, it has been mostly observed during January to March and August to October. The average oestrous cycle in Alsatian bitches is about 150 days and in Boston bitches, it is about 240 days. The different phases of oestrous cycle are the anoestrous, pro-oestrous, oestrous and metoestrous.

i) Mating behaviour of bitches

Bitches in kennels and pet bitches do not have choice and mated to assigned stud. Rarely any breeding problem is observed in pet dogs. However, mating behaviour of stray dogs is quite different. A stray bitch is followed by almost all eligible stray dogs of the locality or group inhabiting the area, lane or street but dominant male keeps all other males away, indeed pups of varying phenotypes are born in most of the cases and it is generally easy to identify the sire(s). However, it is not uncommon to find exceptional mating. By close observation of litters of several stray bitches, one can find a bitch with identical pups in the litter, an indicator of monogamy. At times rare incidence of mating may be observed in stray bitches that mates with a male outside the group.

Eloping is frequently observed in pet bitches. It is very difficult to confine a bitch in heat. A little lapse in controlling is enough for escaping. Mating in eloped bitches is very quick as on search within few minutes she is found tied with male.

ii) The Gestation or Pregnancy

Bitches are ready for conception after 6-9 months of age in different breeds but breeding is allowed at 9-12 month of age and at 3rd or 4th oestrous. Gestation period may range from 55 to 66 days (average 63 days) in different breeds.

iii) The Pseudopregnancy or Fantum Pregnancy

Appearance of signs of pregnancy without mating is frequently observed in bitches. It appears after puberty during the luteal phase of oestrous. The reason is considered to be hormonal imbalance inhibiting the regression of corpus luteum. The signs become visible with the increase in abdominal dimension due to deposition of fat and development of mammary glands. There may be odourless mucous discharge from the vulva and some bitches also start nest making and behave like a true pregnant bitch approaching parturition. The condition may lost full term of normal pregnancy. Variation in rate of pseudopregnancy is very high and it ranges from 3 to 40 per cent in different breeds. The condition can be treated by hormone therapy in known cases of pet bitches in the house.

4.15 Pregnancy Diagnosis in Bitch

Following changes in the behaviour and body of the bitch provides satisfactory diagnosis of pregnancy:

1. A significant reduction in aggressiveness and physical activities by the middle of gestation period.
2. Craving for more food and increased liking for bone gnowing.
3. Gradual increase in letharginess from sixth of gestation period.
4. Progressing increase in abdomen after 5-6 weeks of pregnancy. This occurs due to faster growth of litter, associated foetal membranes and fluid, and also the deposition of adipose tissue during the period.

5. The mammary glands are differentiated by an imaginary line on either side on the abdomen after 6 weeks of pregnancy. The udder becomes prominently enlarged and oedematous. The teats are prominent due to enlargement and turgidity. The mammary system appears smooth and bright during the terminal days of pregnancy.
6. The stray bitches search a safe place for whelping while pet bitches start nest making by collecting papers, cotton and clothes. Hairy and double coated bitches pool their body coat for making nest. In kennels, adequate bedding is provided.
7. The increase in size of abdomen should be differentiated from pseudopregnancy and asctes.

4.16 Signs of Approaching Whelping

1. The bitch approaching whelping seeks isolation at a lonely and safe place.
2. She stops eating about 8-10 hours before the start of whelping.
3. The external genitalia is swollen due to engorgement and there is a thick and clear mucous discharge from the genital tract.
4. The bitch is initially restless and then lies on sides at the start of labour pain.

   In normal condition, whelping starts after 3-5 waves of labour pain and first pup is delivered. Bitch herself takes care for removal of pup sac and also cuts unbroken naval cord. This is followed by expulsion of other puppies in quick succession.

5. If delay in expulsion of first foetus is more than 2 hours, the labour pain may be weak. The bitch may be exhausted due to repeated attemp of delivary. At this stage, veterinarian must be called for the management of safe whelping.

   However, from remote places, it is better to shift the bitch at a safe place. If it is not possible the owner should keep the following medicines and other materials for use in need during parturition: (a) sterilized clean towel, (b) cotton wool, (c) new or boiled blade or scissors,(d) dettol and tincture iodine, (e) cotton thread, (f) ergot preparata, (g) heating arrangement, (h) castor oil and (i) glucose, sugar or jaggery.

4.17 Whelping or Parturition

It is completed in the following four successive stages:

1. Dilatation of cervix and flow of mucous starts. The bitch lies on sides. Water bag comes out of vulva and it ruptures to lubricate the passage.
2. Strong waves of labour pain starts and movement of foetus towards vagina may be seen on the abdomen from a distance.
3. Expulsion of foetus starts and mostly completed in 30-90 minutes.
4. Expulsion of placenta and debris.

4.18 Nursing of the Puppies

The dam give characteristic call and pushes puppies for holding and suckling a teat. Nursing is mostly performed in lying position but it is also common in standing position (See figures in the last of this chapter). Bitches generally feed at short interval of 3-4 hours in beginning which is gradually increased to 5-6 hours in the 8th week of nursing period. The puppies are mostly weaned at 6 to 8 weeks of age.

4.19 Selection and Management of Brood Bitches

Following criteria are used for the selection of brood bitches:

1. It should be true to the breed and should provide ancestory atleast upto grand parents of dam and sire.
2. The look should be feminine and teats should be properly placed from pectoral region to inguinal region.
3. Body condition should be optimum and obesity should not be controlled either by reducing energy intake or increasing the intensity of exercise.
4. Oestrus cycle should be regular and should occur twice annually during the breeding seasons (November-January and July-September).
5. The bitch should be free from diseases particularly the pleuriparous bitches.
6. Bitches failing to conceive from a potent stud should be removed from the breeding programme and may be placed before veterinarians for necessary investigation. Spraying may be opted for infertile females.

4.20 Summary of Reproduction in Bitch and Queen (female cat)

The events of reproduction in bitch are presented with that of queen (female cat) with the aim of providing some important values of cat which is gaining popularity in Indian houses of many cities (Table 1):

Table 1. Reproductive events in Bitch and Queen (Female Cat)

Reproductive events	Bitch	Queen (Female cat)
Age at puberty (months)	6-12 (7-10)	6-15 (8-10)
Age at first breeding (months)	12-18	12-18
Number of oestrous cycle per year	1-4 (2)	Polyoestrous at 15-21 days
Diameter of mature follicle (mm)	6-8	-
Oestrous duration (days)	4-13 (8-10)	9-10 (4-6)
Time of ovulation	1-2 days after the onset of true oestrus.	24-30 hours after (27) coitus.
Optimum time of mating	2-3 days after true oestrous.	
Transport of ovum (days)	6-8	4-8
Nursing duration (weeks)	6-8	
Suggestion for next breeding	3-4 weeks post Weaning or first oestrous.	First oestrous or next oestrous.

NB: Elopement of queen in eat is quite common.

Stray bitch may be seen surrounded by eligible male dogs with the start of proestrous.

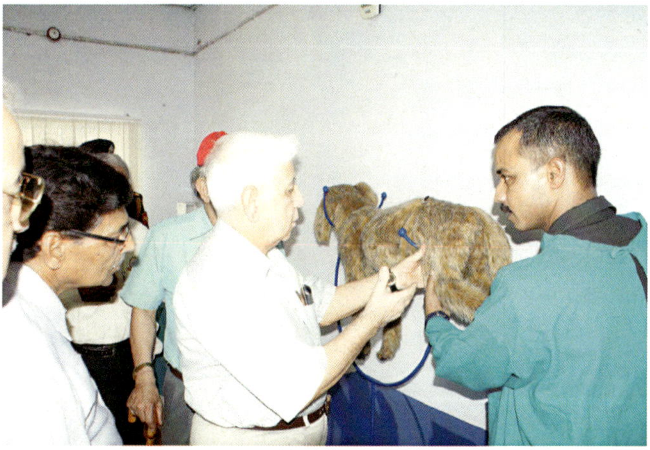

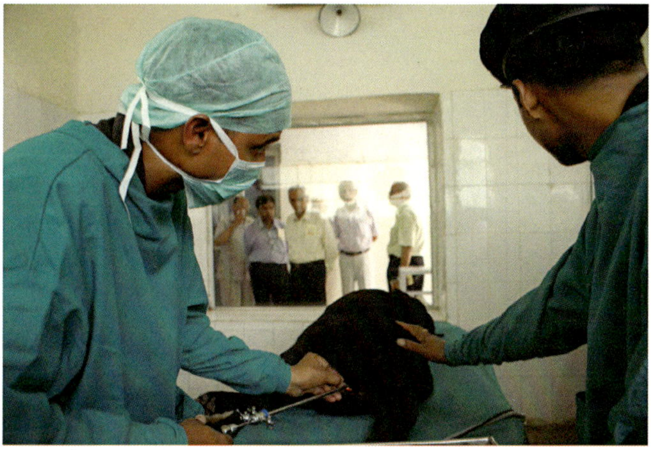

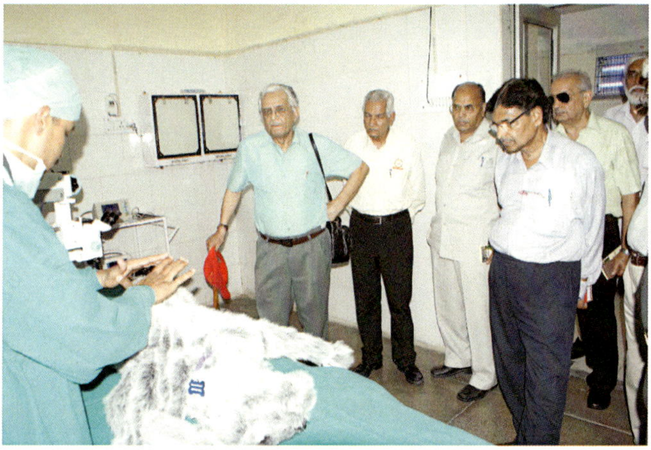

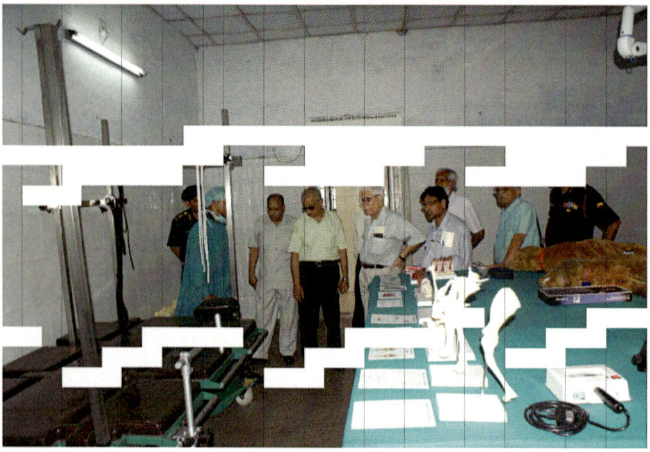

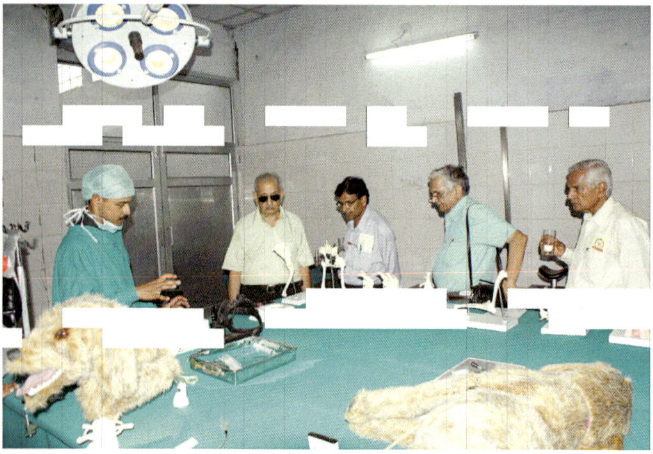

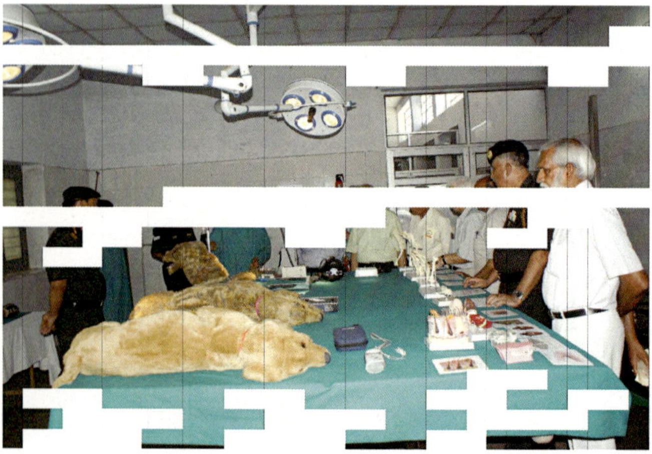

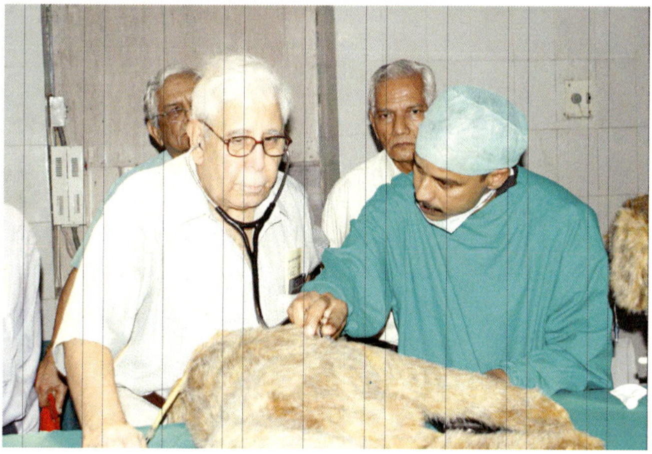

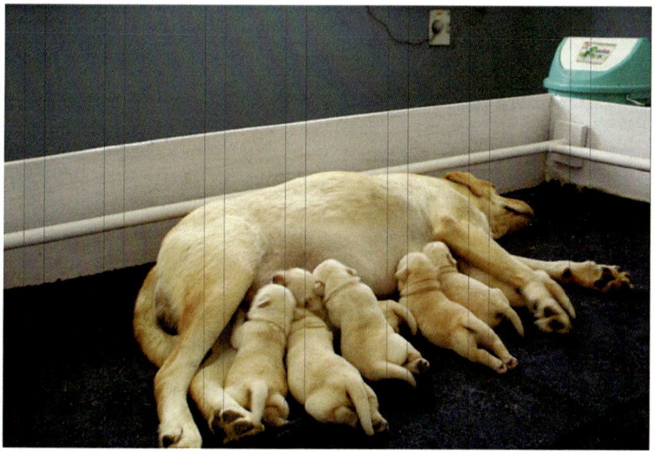

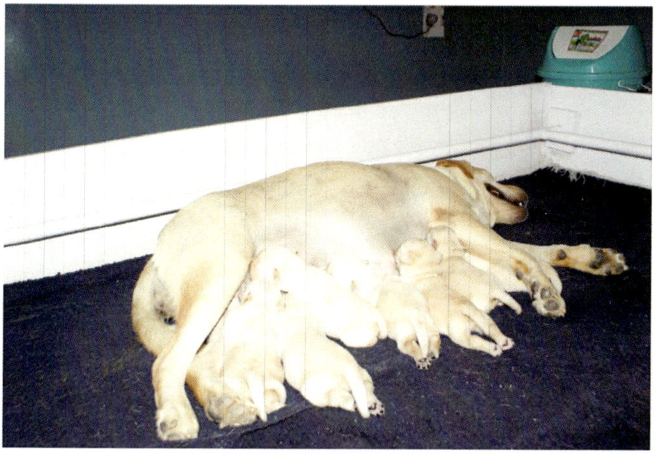

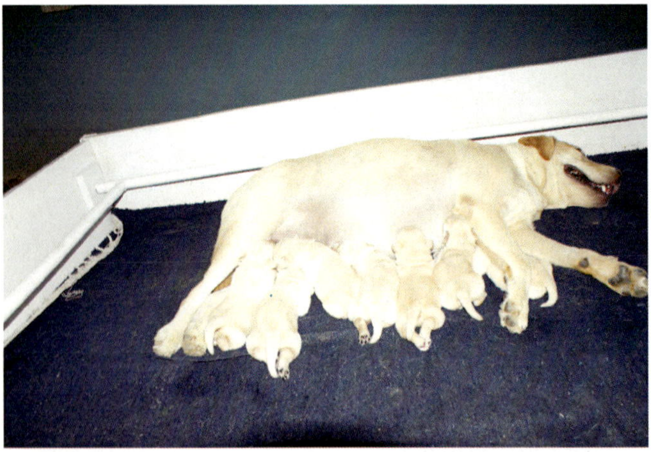

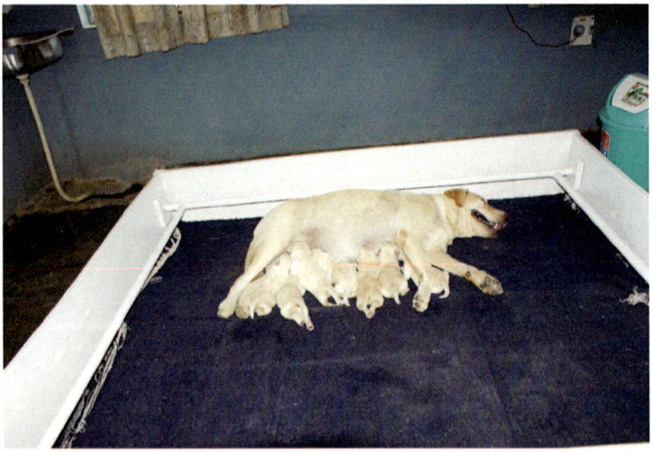

□□□

Chapter 5

Digestive System of Dog, Digestion and Metabolism

5.1 Introduction

The dog is a carnivorous animal by evolution which has been made omnivorous to greater extent after domestication and also complete vegetarian including milk and milk products in the families of strict vegetarian people of India. These changes in the food habits of dogs after domestication have brought some physical changes in the gastrointestinal tract of the dogs reared on carbohydrate rich fibrous diets. The volume of large intestine has increased in the stray dogs of India which feed mostly on the garbage and kitchen let over of hotels, restaurants and dhabas, etc. Despite of all such physical changes, the digestive system of dogs remained simple. The digestive system of dog is as usual a tubuloglandular organ extending from the mouth to terminate at the anus. This has different structural and functional modifications for specific functions like biting, prehension, chewing, swallowing, digestion, absorption of digested portion of foods and defecation. The digestive ystem of dog is differentiated into the mouth or oral cavity, pharynx, oesophagus, stomach, small intestine and large intestine opening through anus.In addition, there are important accessory organs like liver, gall bladder, pancreas and spleen actively involved in digestion and absorption of nutrients. There is great variation in the size of digestive system due to large variation in body size. In this chapter, size of a medium dog of 20 to 30 kg body weight has been taken representative.

5.2 The Mouth or Oral Cavity

The shape and size of oral cavity ranges from short and broad as in boxer and bull dog breeds to long and wide in mastiff breeds and long and narrow in greyhound, Rampur houns, saluki and Whippet, etc. The oral cavity is formed of: (i) the rima oris, (ii) the lips or buccae,

(iii) the cheeks, (iv) the hard palate, (v) the soft palate, (vi) the tongue and (vii) the teeth.

The rima oris or boundary of the oral cavity is very extensive and the labial commissures often extend beyond the level of third cheek teeth. The two sensitive and thin lips are mobile. There are many tactile hairs which are more on the upper lip. A small and distinct bare area on the central part of the upper lip is more sensitive. It also possesses a central depression called the philtrum. In bulldog, this philtrum is more deep and may create confusion for hare lip, if not observed closely. The upper lip in some of the heavy breeds develops in a heavy flew. The flabby border of lower lip is serrated in most of the breeds. The mucous membrane of the buccal cavity is generally pigmented and defined frena labiorum is formed. Scattered small labial glands are scanty.

The voluminous and flaccid cheeks is lined with smooth and usually pigmented mucous membrane on either side at the level of third upper pre-molar tooth. Salivary glands drain in the mouth at different places. A group of four or five ducts of zygomatic glands open on either side at the level of the last molar tooth. The ventral buccal glands are placed against the cheek teeth in series with interior labial glands. The anterior portion of upper oral cavity forms the hard palate which is divided into two lateral halves by a shallow some-times in distinct median raphe. The mucosa of hard palate is folded in 8 to 10 curved transverse ridges on either side of the median raphe. The hard palate is widest at the level of last pair of the pre-molar to firsy pair of the molar teeth. A blunt triangular papilla incisive is present behind the first pair of upper incisor teeth and on this papilla naso-paletine (incisive) ducts drain. As usual mucous membrane of hard palate is also pigmented. The hard palate extends posteriorly to form soft palate which is thick in the central part and thinner laterally. It comes in contact with the epiglottis, when the animal is at rest otherwise the epiglottis remains ventral. A well-developed tonsillar sinus on either side is situated between the anterior and posterior pillars of the soft palate. The long fusiform tonsil is present in the tonsillar sinus. The pinkish red tonsil of about 25 mm is present entirely enclosed in the two-folds of the mucous membrane. The posterior pillar of the soft palate is double of which upper fold extends just with the upper wall, whereas lower fold fuses with the sides of epiglottis.

5.3 The Tongue

The tongue is unpigmented bright pinkish red muscular and spoon shaped. It is broad and thin anteriorly and gradually becomes thicker posteriorly. It always remains wet in healthy dogs. The tongue is highly mobile and mostly remains protruded during most of the time particularly during the hot season. The dorsal surface (dorsum) of the tongue possesses a median groove called sulcus medianus linguae. The dorsum is also covered with a thick layer of posteriorly directed short filiform papillae. On the root of the tongue, there are posteriorly pointing long and soft conical papillae. Such papillae are also present on the labial walls of the isthmus faucium. Another fungi form papillae are present scattered on the dorsum and sides of the tongue. However, these are not found in the area of conical papillae extending to posterior part of the dorsum and root of the tongue. At the place of the beginning of conical papillae, a set of two or three valate papillae are found on either side of the posterior part of dorsum. Oval shaped foliate papillae crossed by fine fissures are present in front of the anterior pillars on the soft palate. A fusiform cord like structure called lyssa is found on the ventral aspect of tip of the tongue. The lyssa is composed of muscles, fibrous tissue and adipose tissue, and its length may be 2 to 5 cm in different breeds depending on the size of dog. The tongue is main organ of prehension in dogs and only organ for the intake of liquid.

5.4 The Teeth or Dento

The teeth are specialized bony structures of different shape, size and strength arranged in a well-defined order. These are present embedded in gum on either jaw. The tooth is formed of a small white crown, a defined neck and the long root (forked in cheek teeth) fixed in sockets on each gum. The incisor teeth are present almost vertical on both jaws and their size increases from the central pair to lateral pair. The crown of incisors possess three projections, of which central one is largest. Slightly concave lingual surface two types of teeth are found in the dogs. The initial milk or deciduous teeth are temporary which are replaced by the permanent teeth. As shown in the following dental formulae:

a) Milk/decicuous/temporary teeth dI 3/3 dC 1/1 dP 3/3 dM 0/0 = 28

b) Permanent teeth pI 3/3 pC 1/1 pP 4/4 pM 2/3 = 42

Total number of permanent teeth is normally 42 (20/22) but in some short head (brachycephalus) breeds the number of cheek teeth may be less than normal 13 (6+7). The reduced number of cheek teeth is usually 12 (5+7) but in some extremely rare case, the cheek teeth may be 9 (4 +5) resulting to total 34 teeth. Normally decrease in number of cheek teeth is equal on either jaw but in some exceptional dog reduction in teeth may be unilateral.

i) Eruption pattern of teeth

Eruption of teeth is time taking and often create problem in eating. Most of the dogs avoid hard food during the eruption of teeth. Normal eruption pattern of temporary and permanent teeth is presented in Table 1.

Table 1. Normal teeth eruption pattern in dogs.

Tooth type	Deciduous/Milk/ Temporary	Permanent
Incisors 3 pair on each jaws	4 to 5 weeks	4 to 5 months
Canine 1 pair on both jaws	3 to 5 weeks	4 to 5 months
Pre-molars on both jaws:		
1st pair	4 to 5 months	5 to 6 months
2nd pair	4 to 5 months	do
3rd & 4th pairs	3 to 4 months	do
Molars:		
1st pair	Absent	4 months
2nd upper pair	Absent	5 to 6 months
2nd lower pair	Absent	4 to 5 months
3rd pair (lower only)	Absent	6 to 7 months

The incisor teeth are arranged almost vertical on both the jaws and their size increases from the central pair to lateral pair. The crown of the incisors possesses three projections, of which central one is largest. Slightly concave lingual surface and the corresponding convex labial surface is distinguished from the neck by the cingulum (a V shaped ridge). The narrow roots are deeply fixed in the sockets on jaws. The upper incisors are larger in size than the corresponding lower ones and may be placed scissors bite or level (pinscher bite). In some very rare cases, there may be one or two supernumerary teeth.

The canine teeth are larger with pointed conical crown. The labial surface is prominently convex and lingual surface is concave. A considerable gap is present between the lateral incisor and the canine tooth of the upper jaw, in which crown of the lower canine tooth rests in the closed mouth. The laterally flattened root is fixed deeper in the jaws.

The cheek teeth are mostly 26 [2(6 + 7)] in number. These include 4 pre-molars and 2 molars on the upper jaw, and 4 pre-molars and 3 molars on the lower jaw. In some breeds with brachycephalic face, the number of cheek teeth is mostly less (5/7 or in some case even 4/5). The fourth pair on upper jaw and fifth pair on lower jaw are largest cheek teeth and called sectorial or carnassic teeth.

5.5 The Salivary Glands

Four types of salivary glands open in the mouth of dogs. These are parotid, mandibular, sublingual and zygomatic glands. The parotid glands are small and irregular. A duct from each parotid gland opens at the level of third upper pre-molar tooth. In some rare dogs, there may be accessory parotid glands. The mandibular glands are somewhat round, pale, encapsulated and larger than the parotid glands. The mandibular glands open on a rudimentary papilla present near the frenum linguae.

The sublingual gland is pink colour and placed close to mandibular gland and opens either near the opening of mandibular gland or joins it to drain together. The zygomatic gland is situated on the anterior aspect of the pterygo-palatine fossa. The gland opens through 4 or 5 ducts at the level of the last molar tooth.

5.6 The Pharynx

It is a junction of oral cavity, larynx and Eustachian tubes. The slit like opening of latter is regulated by round shape projection of mucous membrane, which is known as torus tubarius.

5.7 The Oesophagus

The musculo-epithelial tubular part of the alimentary canal starts as a relatively narrower continuation of oral cavity from the constricted isthmus oesophagi and joins the stomach. A thin layer of tubulo-alveolar mucous glands are present on its ventral surface. The oesophagus is formed of two spiral layers of striated muscles, which are arranged in longitudinal and circular muscle near the cardia.

5.8 The Stomach

It is a relatively larger musculo-glandular sac of irregular shape, when full. The shape is piriform. The outer greater curvature of stomach is much longer than the lesser curvature. The oesophagus opens in the cardiac part, which extends as the largest fundic part (fundus gland region of the stomach) and the terminal narrower pyloric region. The stomach is hold in position with the help of greater and lesser momentum.

5.9 The Intestines

The intestines of dogs are much shorter and less voluminous than the intestines of herbivorous animals of same size. The length of entire intestine is about five times of the body length from crown to root of the tail. The intestines are differentiated into two types, mainly on the basis of the diameter of lumen and some difference in functions. The anterior part of narrower lumen is called small intestine and the posteior broader part is called large intestine.

The small intestine: It extends from the pylorus and its first elongated U-shaped region is known as duodenum. The remaining longer portion extends in the form of many coils and the terminal ilium portion joins the colon through ilio-colic orifice. The small intestine is hold in position by mesentery.

The large intestine: The large intestine is identified into caecum, colon and rectum. The first two segments are the main areas of absorption while the last segment is the store for the undigested food and secretary wastes. At the junction of rectum with the anus may anal glands present in the squamous epithelium layer. On either side anal glands open through two small openings. These anal sacs (Sinus paranales) contain dirty grey fatty secretion emitting characteristic offensive odour. In the vicinity of anal sac, there are large sebaceous glands and specialized circumanal glands. The opening of anus is controlled by strong sphincters that open only after receiving signal for defecation.

5.10 Accessory Digestive Organs

The glandular accessory organs playing very important roles in the digestion of foods and absorption of nutrients are the liver, pancreas and spleen.

i) The Liver

The average size of liver in dogs is about 3 per cent of the adult body weight. The liver contains five lobes, *viz.* left lateral lobe, left central lobe, right central lobe, right lateral lobe and caudate lobe. The parietal surface of liver is convex, whereas visceral surface is irregularly concave due to depressions formed by the pressure of different organs placed in close contact. The liver parenchyma is formed of polygonal cells and the entire gland is encapsulated in the fibrous tunica serosa. The hepatic duct opens in the duodenum. The gall bladder is a somewhat pear-shaped sac made for the storage of bile. The cystic duct joins the hepatic duct just before opening into the duodenum. The duct opens at some distance from the pylorus.

ii) The Pancreas

This is an irregular V-shaped organ formed of two long and narrow parts. Normally, there are one short and another long pancreatic duct. The short one opens into the duodenum either with bile duct or close to it, while the longer opens a little posterior into the small intestine. The endocrine or secretary cells contain zymogen granules, which are responsible for enzyme production.

iii) The Spleen

The folciform, long and narrow spleen with wide ventral part is red to bright red in colour. The shape and position except ots dorsal end are variable. The main function of spleen is the production of lymphocytes in post natal life but it may also produce erythrocytes, granulocytes and megakaryocytes in the emergency. The spleen plays important role in the formation of bile pigments, storage of iron and some metabolism activities.

5.11 Digestion, Absorption & Metabolism

i) Antibody absorption in neonate puppies

Antibody transfer in dogs is both pre-natal and post-natal for 1-2 days in colostrums, and the contribution of two channels is almost equal. Adsorption of antibodies through the wall of small intestine is a type of endocytosis by the adsorption cells of microvilli. After deposition of antibodies at the border of microvillous, the membrane is invaginated to form vesicles. This process needs additional energy for the replacement of cells of mucosa of microvilli. These vesicles are called phagomes which migrate to supranuclear zone of the cell. At this place, phagosomes fuse with lysosomes to form phagolysosomes. Intracellular digestion occurs in the vesicles but a small part of macromolecules of antibodies escape digestion and migrate to the basolateral surface of the cell membrane. At this point, exocytosis occurs and macromolecules of antibodies enter into the lymphatic system through intercellular space.

ii) Relative capacity of alimentary canal of dog

The mean proportion of stomach, small intestine, caecum and colon including rectum are about 62, 23, 1.5 and 13.5 per cent, respectively. However, composition of diets during the growth phase may alter the ratio to limited extent.

iii) Prehension

The organs of prehension in dogs are the teeth and forelegs (specially paws). Deglutition of food is accomplished by coordinated action of teeth, tongue, jaws and hard palate. Tongue is the only organ for the ingestion of water and other liquids.

iv) Mastication or chewing

The food in mouth is teared mechanically by the incisor teeth and ground by the cheek teeth by vertical movements of jaws. Grinding is mostly incomplete. Saliva is mixed with the food during mastication for proper lubrication to facilitate smooth passage of food bolus through pharynx and oesophagus to stomach.

v) Deglutition or swallowing

Deglutition is a co-ordinated action of different oral organs to cardia in the stomach. The action is initiated by the fast movements of jaws and tongue after the intake of food in the mouth, which subsequently becomes a reflex action during functioning. The ground food is made into a bolus by mixing saliva. The bolus is pushed by the tongue to the poarerior end of the oral cavity. Now, it is pushed into the oesophagus by contraction of the mylohyoid by pressing the tongue against the hard palate and the hyoglossus muscles by drawing the base of tongue backwards. This increases the intrapharyngeal pessure. This is followed by sudden relaxation of the pharyngoesophageal junction controlled by a sphincter like mechanism. Now the food bolus is transported by peristaltic movements of the oesophageal muscles. In dogs, total oesophagus is made of striated muscle fibres.

The salivated food entering through cardia into the fundic part of stomach is stored for gradual transfer into the corpus region for the mixing of gastric juice with the salvated ingesta by churning. The churned ingesta or chyme gradually flows down to antrum and then pushed through pylorus into duodenum. The flow of fluid fraction is faster than the relatively thicker portion . The rate of gastric emptying of cereal foods is faster than the meat based foods. The digestion of carbohydrates and proteins (not the fat) is initiated in the stomach.

The flow of chyme from stomach to small intestine is regulated in a manner to facilitate the mixing of digesta with pancreatic juice containing different hydrolytic enzymes and bile for the digestion of carbohydrates, proteins and lipids and also, the maximum contact of digesta with the mucosa for the greater absorption of nutrients liberated by digestion. The remaining digesta passes into the large intestine for microbial digestion in addition to carry over digestion of carbohydrates and proteins. Contribution of microbial digestion is meager in the dogs. Absorption of electrolytes and water occurs in the large intestine. The faeces is collected in the rectum for periodic avacuation from the body.

vi) Defecation

It is the process of expulsion of undigested food alongwith other waste materials of digestion. In natural state, it is involuntary but has become voluntary to greater extent due to domestication. Normally, 7-10 hours are required for the travel of food from mouth to rectum.

5.12 Functions of Saliva

1. The main functions of saliva are moistening to facilitate mastication and lubrication for easy passage of food bolus across the oesophagus via pharynx.
2. Another important function specially in hot season is the evaporative cooling. The tongue protrudes out during the hot season to expose larger surface for evaporation. The tongue is kept wet by continuous secretion of parotid saliva, which may increase 10 times or even more during the hot climate.

i) Composition of Saliva

The main contents of saliva are sodium in bicarbonates, chloride and potassium in descending order of concentration. It also contains protein but no enzyme.

5.13 Functions of Gastric Juice

The mucosa of stomach is differentiated into cardiac, gastric and pyloric regions. The largest area of stomach is covered by gastric mucosa, which secrets pepsinogen (pro pepsin) and hydrochloric acid (HCl). Only small amount of mucous is secreted by the small area of cardiac mucosa.

5.14 Functions of Exocrine Secretions of Pancreas

1. Secretion of bicarbonate ions (HCO_3) reduces the acidity of digesta entering into the duodenum. ($HCl + NaHCO_3 = NaCl + CO_2 + H_2O$).
2. **Secretion of pancreatic enzymes:** This contains all the essential enzymes required for the digestion of carbohydrates, proteins and lipids.
   a) Protease is secreted in an inactive form trypsinogen, which is converted into active trypsin. This reaction is initially inhibited in the pancreas for its protection from the digestive action of trypsin. Trypsinogen is converted to active trypsin form by the enterokinase secreted in the small intestine. The intestinal secretion is called succus entericus.

   b) Pancreatic amyase is secreted in an active form and hydrolyses the greater proportion of ingested carbohydrates in absorbable smaller molecules of simple sugars.

c) Dietary fats (triglycerides) are hydrolysed by the action of pancreatic lipase.

The enzyme is activated by bile acids for the solubilization of end products and formation of micelles. The reaction requires more than 2mm concentration of bile acids in the jejunal part of the small intestine.

d) Digestion of fat occurs only in small intestine but that of carbohydrates and proteins continues in large intestines.

5.15 Synthesis of Bile

1. Bile salts are synthesized in the hepatocytes from cholesterol.
2. Bile acids produced cholic acid and some amount of chenoleoxycholic acid, which conjugate with taurine or glycine.

5.16 Digestion and Absorption of Carbohydrates in the Small Intestine

1. **Luminal digestion:** It occurs in the lumen of small intestine by the action of pancreatic alpha-amylase on the dietary starch. The hydrolysates are mainly disaccharides (maltose), some amount of trisaccharides (trimaltose and some branched chain oligosaccharides). These molecules are not absorbed.
2. **Mucosal digestion and absorption:** The disaccharides and trisaccharides come in contact with the mucosa of small intestine and further hydrolyzed by the sacchridases of brush border of the intestinal mucosa to produce monosaccharides that are transported into the portal vein for diffusion in the body for further utilization for the supply of energy.

5.17 Digestion and Absorption of Proteins in Small Intestine

Pepsin hydrolysis of proteins starts in the stomach after the converssion of pepsinogen into active pepsin but main digestion occurs in the upper part of small intestine in three phases, *viz.* (i) hydrolysis of proteins occurs by the action of pancreatic peptidases. Two groups of inactive pancreatic peptidases are discharged in the duodenum. These pro-enzymes are endopeptidases comprising of trypsinogen, chymotrypsinogen and slastase. The others are carboxypeptidases A and B-These pro-enzymes are activated by the enterokinase at the brush border of the intestinal mucosal cells.

Trypsinogen is activated by enerokinase to form trypsin which subsequently activates the other pro-enzymes. The hydrolysates of pancreatic proteases are the neutral and basic amino acids and oligopeptides. Smaller oligopeptides formed of less than 6 amino acids accumulate in the intestinal contents and then hydrolysed at the brush border to facilitate absorption. Amino acids and short peptides of two or three amino acids are only absorbed across the intestinal wall.

Absorption of amino acids into the epithelial cells takes place by different specialized systems:

a) Transportation of neutral amino acids,

b) Transportation of basic amino acids,

c) Transportation of dipeptides, and

d) Transportation of tripeptides.

The dipeptides and tripeptides are hydrolyzed to amino acids in the epithelial cells of the small intestine. Indeed about 10 per cent absorbed peptides escape hydrolysis and enter circulation. However, these are not utilized in the body and excreted in urine.

5.18 Digestion and Absorption of Fat

The dietary fats are largely water insoluble triglycerides that are emulsified in the stomach. The passage of emulsified fat molecules into the duodenum is a controlled mechanism for providing sufficient time for its digestion performed by co-ordinated action of pancreatic secretion and bile. Pancreatic lipase disintegrate the fat molecules into beta-monoglyceride and two molecules of fatty acids. These products are also not soluble in water. These are known as amphipaths means a part is polar and water soluble and remaining part is non-polar and fat soluble.

The solubilization of these products is facilitated by the detergent action of bile acids and negative charged micelles are formed. These micelles are the actual carrier of fat molecules across the intestinal mucosa. The micelles capture the water insoluble substance and dissolve. For the formation of micelle, the concentration of bile acids in the jejunum should be more than 2 mm. This is known as critical miceller concentration of bile acids. The conversion of fat from an emulsion to micelle, the diameter of particles is reduced almost 100 times and surface area increase is more than 10,000 times. Micelles carry the fatty acids to brush border of the intestinal epithelial cells.At this place, fat is released that diffuse through the lipid membrane into the cell content.

In the epithelial cells, the fatty acids and monoglycerides are again esterified to form cellular triglycerides. After these join cholesterol, cholesterol esters, phospholipids and a small quantity of protein to form chylomicrons. These chylomicrons transport the water insoluble fats. Coating of protein is essential for the transportation of triglycerides inside the body tissues.

i) Digestion and Absorption in Large Intestine

Digestion in large intestine is carried by the enzymes synthesized by the normal micro-organism inhabiting large intestine. The little soluble and all fibrous carbohydrates are metabolized to produce volatile fatty acids (acetic, propionic and butyric), small amount of lactic acid, carbon dioxide, methane and water. The environment of large intestine is maintained by the two buffer (bi-carbonate and phosphate) systems because slow absorption rate of volatile fatty acids (VFA) is very slow that reduces the pH of the contents in large intestine.

Undigested residual dietary protein entering the large intestine is digested by microbial enzymes to produce amino acids, small peptides and ammonia. Only ammonia is absorbed in the body to be eliminated in urine. There appears to be no information on the further utilization of amino acids and peptides, and it is excreted in the faeces.

5.19 Intermediary Metabolism

This is most important step in the utilization of nutrients for different functions in the body after these are transported into the body system from the foods digested in the alimentary canal.

i) Carbohydrate Metabolism

Monosaccharides (largely glucose) absorbed in blood are quickly transported into liver and then into general circulation. Other monosaccharides in small quantity are also transformed into glucose in liver.

ii) Functions of Liver in Carbohydrate Metabolism

1. Other monosaccharides (fructose and galactose) are transformed into glucose.
2. Glycogenesis.
3. Glycogenolysis.
4. Gluconeogenesis.
5. Conversion of carbohydrates into fats.

iii) Fate of Blood Glucose

1. Utilization of glucose by tissue cells for energy.
2. Storage of glucogen in the form of glycogen (Animal starch) mainly in muscles and traces in other cells. Glycogen is utilized by glycolysis to yield pyruvic acid. The pyruvic acid is metabolized to CO_2 and H_2O in the presence of oxygen, but in the deficit oxygen, pyruvic acid is converted to lactic acid.

5.20 Summary of Metabolism of Glucose, FFA, Triglycerol and Amino Acids

Foods digested

↕

Nutrients absorbed (Organic part)

↕

Glucose	Free fatty acids	Triglycerols	Amino acids	
			↕	

↕	↕	↕	↕	
			Ammonia	
			↕	
			Urea	Protein
Used for energy, Glycogen, fatty acid and triglyceride	Triglycerols -------- Used for energy, triglyceride and fatty acid synthesis		↕	↕ Amino acids

Chapter 6

Foods of Dogs and Nutrients Supply

6.1 Foods

All kinds of organic and inorganic substances eaten by the animals for the supply of nutritional requirement of body for maintaining normal physiological functions are known as foods. The foods should also provide satiety. These are mostly natural products but may be synthetic also. Synthetic foods are generally micro nutrients like minerals and vitamins supplemented in small quantity for balancing the diets. The term, food, is primarily used for the human foods. This term has been adopted for the nutrition of few simple stomached animals like dogs, cats and primates fed similar foods.

6.2 Main Functions of Foods

The functions of foods may be put in the following broad categories:

1. Formation of tissue for growth and repaire due to wear and tear.
2. Synthesis of enzymes and incretions.
3. Strenthening of immune system (antibodies) for providing protection against infectious diseases.
4. Balancing of nutrients supply for protection against nutritional disorders caused by deficiency and imbalance of nutrients.
5. Metabolism of organic foods for the liberation of energy to maintain body temperature, work and regulation of heat production during hot and cold season.
6. **Satiety:** It is the state of feeling freedom from hunger due to ingestion of enough food. Sometimes, it is considered that any substance entering the stomach can produce satiety, but it is not true.

6.3 Composition of Foods for Dogs

The dogs are carnivorous by evolution and in wild conditions they eat carcass of kills, residual cadaver hunted by other wild animals or dead carcass.Though the dogs are carnivorous animals by evolution, but in the process of domestication, they have adapted well the omnivorous feeding. In many Indian families of strict vegetarians, the pet dogs are reared in optimum health condition with little milk feeding in early life. Normal diets of dogs include the foods of plant and animal origin, and may require supplementation of micro nutrients, which are mostly synthetic chemicals. Following are the common sources of foods:

1. **Foods of plant origin**: The foods of plant origin:
   a) Starchy cereal grains like rice, wheat, maize, pearl millet, sorghum, pearled barley, pearled oats, finger millet, paspalum and other minor millets.
   b) The pulses and leguminous seeds are moderate sources of carbohydrates and proteins, and include gram, pea, lentil, pigeon pea, green bean, black bean, soyabean and kidney bean, etc.
   c) The oilseeds are rich sources of lipids and moderate sources of proteins and carbohydrates and include linseed, sesame seeds, groundnut, canola seed, soybeans, sunflower seeds and safflower seeds.
   d) The oilseed extractions (cakes) like groundnut cake, linseed cake, soyabean meal, sunflower seed cake, sesame cake and others.
   e) Cereals and pulses milling byproducts like wheat bran, broken rice, fresh rice polish, broken pulses including embryos and some hulls.
   f) The other foods of plant origin are the roots and tubers like potatoes, sweet potato, carrot, beets, turnip and cassava, etc. The fruits are mango, litchi, banana, guava, papaya, sapota, orange, apple, pears and all other fruits eaten by humans.
   g) All kinds of vegetables like spinach, amaranthus, cabbage and water spinach are also used in the diets of dogs.
   h) Fruits like mango, guava, litchi, pomegranate, custard apple, apple, pears, sapota, pine apple, plum, grapes, papaya, etc.

2. **Foods of animal origin:** These include :

   a) Sources of edible flesh like beef, buffen, mutton, chevon, pork, lights and poultry. These generally include carcass trimmings, lights, glands, etc.

   b) Aquatic creatures like shortings of fishes, crab, lobster, snails and unio, etc.

   c) Milk and milk products of all domesticated mammalian species, and eggs of poultry birds and turtoise.

3. **Food supplements**: These are mostly synthetic chemicals like minerals, vitamins and some essential amino acids. These are used in small quantity for balancing the diets of different physiological stages. Such supplementation is more needed in vegetarian diets.

4. **Food additives**: These are usually non-nutrient substances used in small quantity for stimulating the performance and also, the development of body resistence. Some modern additives are called nutraceuticals and herbiceuticals. These include fibrous carbohydrates, spices, plant extracts, etc.

5. **Colours and flavours:** These are harmless natural or synthetic substances used for the improvement of appearance and palatability of the prepared foods. These are generally used in commercial foods.

   Foods not to be fed without heat treatment.

Many raw foods anti-nutritional factors that interfere in digestibility and availability of nutrients. There are some harmful foods, when fed raw. Some of such foods are listed as follows:

1. Raw milk of dairy animals.
2. Raw eggs.
3. Uncooked soyabean and other legumes.
4. Raw flesh and bones.
5. Raw fish and also cooked fish containing spicules.
6. Feeding of blood in any form should be avoided.
7. Spoiled foods.

6.4 Nutrients

The nutrients supply from the diets determine the health and performances of dogs. For optimum physiological functions, a balanced blend of nutrients is essential. The six important groups of basic essential nutrients are water, carbohydrates, lipids, proteins, minerals and vitamins. The carbohydrates and lipids are the main sources of energy but excess of dietary protein intake is also utilized for energy supply, but during energy deficiency in the body either due to clinicopathological causes or due to starvation, the body's issue protein is mobilized for the energy supply for maintaining the vital functions for survival.

6.5 Water

Regular supply of drinking water is essential for the survival and normal physiological functions of the body. Water constitutes more than 60% of the body mass. It is maximum in infants and gradually decreases with the increase in age. Water content is also less in the body of obese dogs. Deprivation of water causes dehydration resulting in the occurrence of several clinical conditions. Severe dehydration may be fatal on delayed rehydration.

Functions of water in the body: Followings are some of the important functions of water in the body:

1. Essential for the biochemical reactions in the body.
2. Maintenance of fluid (blood, lymph and tissue fluids) volume.
3. Transportation of absorbed nutrients to target organs for vital functions.
4. Elimination of waste metabolites in urine, sweat and faeces.
5. Regulation of body temperature.

Factors affecting water intake: Water intake is influenced by the age, sex, growth, pregnancy, lactation, dry food intake, environmental temperature, humidity, speed of dry air movement and clinical conditions like diarrhoea, dysentery and vomiting, etc.

Sources of water: Drinking water content in foods eaten and metabolic water produced during the metabolism of carbohydrates, fat and protein in the body at the rate of 0.6, 1.1 and 0.4 ml per (g) of metabolized nutrients, respectively.

6.6 Energy

Dietary energy is the functional form of the organic constituents of food. The supply of energy is made by the metabolism of carbohydrates, lipids and proteins intake in the diets. The different methods of energy measurement are used in nutrition are starch equivalent (SE), total digestible nutrient (RDN), gross energy (GE), digestible energy (DE), metabolizable energy (ME) and net energy (NE). The first two are determined as pound (lb) or kilogramme (kg) or gram (g) and the last three are measured as joule (j), kilojoule (kj), megajoule (mj), calorie (cal), kilocalorie (kcal) or megacalorie (mcal). In routine practice, dietary energy is frequently mentioned as calorie that depicts 1 kcal of energy. For all practical feeding only kcal or kj are used in most of the countries and conversion factor is 1 kcal.

Energy provides necessary force for the physiological functions in the body and responsible for the utilization of all the essential nutrients for the maintenance of body, growth, reproduction and production. Average metabolizable energy values of different organic nutrients are as follows:

Carbohydrates	3.5 kcal per g
Proteins	3.5 kcal per g
Fats	8.5 kcal per g

i) Measurement of the energy value of foods

Like all other domestic animals, the dogs are also not capable of utilizing the entire energy content (Gross Energy or GE) of a food or diet. The energy utilized in the body is measured in the following forms:

Gross energy (GE) = It is total energy liberated on complete combustion of 1 gram dry matter of food under the pressure of oxygen gas in a bomb calorimeter.

Digestible energy (DE) = GE intake– GE excreted in faeces. The faeces is the undigested portion of food intake.

Metabolizable Energy (ME) = DE of feed– GE excreted in urine.

Actually ME in a food or diet is available to the animals for performing all kinds of physiological (vital) functions in the body. The requirement of ME depends on the physiological state of the animal and the environmental factors of the habitat.

ii) Factors affecting the energy (calorie) requirement of dogs

Some of the important factors affecting the energy requirement of the dogs are:

1. **Physiological state of the body:** Energy requirement for the maintenance of adult dogs is lowest and it increases two to four folds for supplying the requirements of growing puppies, growing pups, pregnant bitches, nursing bitches, stud dogs and working dogs.
2. **Breed of the dog:** There is large variation in the body weight of different breeds. It ranges from 1 kg to 5 kg in the toy and small breeds to more than 70 kg in the large breeds. Maintenance requirement of adult dogs per unit (kg or lb) body weight slightly decreases with the increase in adult body size. The maintenance energy requirement of growing, pregnant and nursing dogs is also a little more than the idle dogs. However, consideration of these differences in maintenance requirement of productive dogs are included in their requirements for production.

   Daily ME requirement of dogs of less than 10 kg body weight for maintenance is about 110 kcal/kg body weight. It decreases to 65-90 kcal/kg for 10-25 kg body weight and 45-65 kcal/kg body weight for the adult dogs of more than 25 kg body weight.
3. **Effect of physical activities:** Small breeds of dogs are much active than the larger breeds and this factor has been considered in breed effect. The activities may range from light work of guarding the premises to moderate work of controlling the farm animals on pastures, hard work of chasing and catching the games and strenuous work of pulling the sledge in hostile climate. Some estimates of energy requirement for work of different intensity has been worked out with the use of treadmill, but there appears to be no information on the energy requirement of actual working dogs chasing the games and sledge dogs pulling the cart for long distance. Such dogs are mostly fed high energy diets containing greater proportion of fatty tissue. Commercial foods should be enriched with fat, butter or oil so that the dogs may not consume other unnecessary higher amount of other nutrients, particularly protein and minerals.
4. **Effect of season:** Climatic stress increases the requirement of energy. During cold season, more energy is required for keeping

the body warm. In hot season, expenditure of energy increase for dissipating the body heat by panting and during the humid season additional unwanted work is required for repelling the flies, mosquitoes and other ecto-parasites.

5. **Effect of latent wasting diseases:** Energy expenditure for maintenance may increase in clinicopathological condition caused by gastrointestinal parasitism and the chronic wasting diseases.

6.7 Carbohydrates

These constitute the basal diets and main source of energy in the normal diets. These include sugars, starch, cellulose and hemicellulose. The common sources of carbohydrates are the cereal grains like maize, rice, wheat, sorghum, pearl millet, finger millet and paspalum, etc. potatoes, sweet potato, tapioca (cassava), carrot and turnip, etc. The pulses and leguminous seeds also contain moderately high level of protein. Sugars are not utilized efficiently due to lack of sucrases and should not be included in the dog food formulations.

i) Disturbance in carbohydrate digestion and absorption

In many gastrointestinal disorders (diarrhoea, dysentery, flatulence, constipation), complete digestion of dietary carbohydrates is hindered at some intermediate step and absorption is disturbed. Lactase is secreted in nursing puppies and lactase is digested and absorbed but its secretion is highly reduced or ceased due to which many adult dogs are unable to digest milk (particularly lactase) and suffer from loose motion and other digestive disorders. However, replacement of mother milk with milk of other species (cow, buffalo, goat, sheep, etc.) in continuation has been found to be utilized in most of the pet dogs and milk is the only source of animal protein in the diets of pets kept in strict vegeterian families of Indian people.

6.8 Dietary Fibre

It is a poorly digestible carbohydrate complex constituent of vegetable foods. The components of dietary fibre are the cellulose, hemicellulose, lignin, pectin, cutin, gum, mucilages and waxes. The digestive enzymes of dogs are not capable to digest fibre complex. A small pack of cellulose and hemicellulose is digested by the action of microbial enzymes and volatile fatty acids (acetic, propionic and butyric) are produced.

Functions of dietary fibre: Although required in small quantity, dietary fibre plays important role in digestion, maintenance of gut health, reproduction and over all health of the dogs. Important functions of dietary fibre may be listed as follows:

1. Some dietary fibres are hygroscopic and possess high water holding ability. Volume of fibres is also increased significantly due to swelling caused by absorption of water.
2. The water absorption, swelling and water holding properties of the dietary fibre changes the retention time of digesta due to changed rate of passage. This property is utilized for the correction of gastrointestinal disorders.
3. High fibre diet causes stomach distention and controls calorie intake. This fact is used for decreasing energy intake in over weight/obese dogs.
4. High proportion of non-stimulating dietary fibres reduces the rate of passage causing delayed emptying of bowel ultimately resulting in less calorie intake.
5. Dietary fibre reduces rate of passage in case of diarrhoea by absorbing water content of digesta. In case of constipation, dietary fibre stimulates bowel movement by causing distension.
6. Dietary fibre also decreases the digestion and absorption of some nutrients by binding.
7. Fibre can also help in removal of some toxins by binding.
8. Excess intake of dietary fibre causes loose faeces, tympany, large volume of faeces voided, increased defaecation number and various degree of energy starvation.

6.9 Protein

Protein is the another essential nutrient that is required for the body building and several biochemical functions. Actually, the constitutional units, the amino acids are the real factors involved in different vital functions in the body. Actually, proteins are the complex nitrogenous compounds formed of large number of different amino acids grouped to form large molecules. Each protein is formed of a definite number of amino acids linked together in precise combination specific for a kind of protein. The dietary proteins are disintegrated into small peptides and free amino acids by the action of proteases and then transported across the intestinal wall to rich in the body pool for further utilization for the synthesis of body proteins.

Amino acids : About twenty amino acids are used for the synthesis of animal protein and ten amino acids are indispensable (essential). The indispensable amino acids are dietary essential because these are not synthesized in the body or a few synthesized in very small quantity. The essential amino acids are not stored in the body for longer period and regular dietary supply is required. Ten essential amino acids are arginine, histadine, isoleucine, leucine, lysine, methionine, phenylalanine, threonine, tryptophan and valine.

Protein requirement of dogs: The requirement of protein depends on the physiological state of the body, stress, physical activities and condition of the body. Dietary protein requirement of growing, pregnant and nursing animals is much higher than the need of idle adult animals. Dietary protein requirement also increases during the healing of cut wounds, burn wounds and healing of fracture and surgical wounds. Normally, protein content in the diets of growing, pregnant and lactating animals should be about 22%, for working adult dogs should be 18-20%, idle adult dogs 16-18% and obese dogs on low calorie diets should be 14-16% on dry matter basis.

Common sources of dietary protein: These include both plant and animal sources. The common sources of animal protein are milk and milk products (not fat rich products), eggs, poultry, meat, fish and flesh of other aquatic animals. The common sources of vegetable protein are the extraction products of soyabean, groundnut, sesame seeds, linseed, pulses and leguminous green pods.

The diets of pregnant bitches should contain plenty of cooked rice and/or cereal flours balanced with good quality protein and other nutrients. Feeding of non-cereal diets often produces whelping problems and birth of low weight puppies of lowered vitality. The actual role of carbohydrates intake on puppies development during gestation, appears to be not yet known.

6.10 Fats

Fats are the richest source of dietary energy and provide two and quarter times more calories than the dietary carbohydrates and proteins. The fats are triglycerides of saturated and unsaturated fatty acids. Unsaturated fatty acids with double bond at carbon atom 3 and 6 in the carbon chain are called omega 3 and 6, respectively, and considered good for the heart health. Dogs are highly efficient in fat utilization and digestion may be more than 90 per cent. The diets of dogs should contain more that 5% fat and preferably 8-12%. There should be adequate supply of linoleic acid and alpha-linoleic acid in the diets of dogs because they are unable to synthesize.

The essential polyunsaturated fatty acids (PUFA) include arachidonic acid, eicosapentaenoic acid (EPA) and docosahexaenoic acid (DHA). Arachidonic acid is a member of omega-6 family, from which prostaglandins, thromboxane and leukotrienes are derived. The deficiency of prostaglandins may adversely affect many of the metabolic processes and the activities of certain hormones. The EPA and DKA belongs to omega-3 family. The deficiency symptoms of PUFA are scaling, alopecia, seborrhea, poor healing of wounds, immuno-suppression and infertility. Supplementation of adequate PUFA is cardioprotective, useful for the prevention and treatment of cancer, skin diseases, metabolic diseases and wounds.

i) Functions of dietary fat

Following are the important functions of dietary fat in the body:

1. Fats are the concentrated energy foods and supply about 3500 kcal ME per kg of maize, wheat and rice, and 9000 kcal per kg fat.
2. Essential fatty acids are supplied by dietary fat which are essential for maintaining healthy skin and body coat.
3. Fats are carrier of fat soluble vitamins and deficiency may cause various ailments due to deficiency of these vitamins on prolonged feeding of fat free diets.
4. Fats make the diets more palatable for the dogs.
5. Fats are also utilized as lubricant in the body.
6. Fatty acids are impotant constituents of cell membranes and play important role in exchange of nutrients and metabolites.

ii) Effects of dietary fat imbalance

Although fat deficiency in dogs is unusual but may occur in rare cases. It is manifested by dry, dull and coarse body coat. Rough, thickened, flaky and dry skin with patches of alopecia. Wounds may be oozing due to secondary infection of abrasion caused by itching of dry skin.

Excess intake of dietary fat is deposited in the adipose tissue and fat depots in the body ultimately resulting in the development of obesity. Obesity is a disqualification for the working dogs and also predisposes the animals for many systemic dieases particularly that of cardiac system.

6.11 Minerals

Minerals are essential nutrients for the formation, development and maintenance of skeleton system and also, for the maintenance of many vital functions in the body. The essential minerals are differentiated into seven major or micro minerals, *viz.* calcium, phosphorus, magnesium, sodium, potassium, chloride and sulphur; and eight defined micro minerals (iron, copper, zinc, iodine, cobalt, manganese, selenium and molybdenum) besides, some yet to be well studied trace minerals. Almost all the minerals are present in different foods but many times either these are deficient or not available due to presence of some binding factors. There are also some harmful minerals ingested due to their mere presence in the foods. Therefore, it is important to know about the mineral composition of common foods, main roles of different minerals in the body and also, the harmful minerals.

Calcium and Phosphorus: These are the main minerals that provide rigidity to skeletal system. Almost 99 per cent of calcium and 80-85 per cent of phosphorus in the body are the constituents of bones and teeth. For the utilization of these minerals for bone growth, their ratio should be 1:1 to 2:1 alongwith adequate supply of vitamin D_3. Wider ratio between the two minerals may disturb their utilization causing deformities of bones and teeth in growing pups and foetal deformities in pregnant bitches. Bones are also the store house of calcium and phosphorus, and trabeculae are present in dynamic form. In case of deficiency, these minerals are mobilized to maintain blood homoeostasis. High calcium in the diet also reduces the absorption of zinc through the intestine.

Other functions of Calcium: It is an essential component of cell content and other body fluids. It is needed for the normal functions of several enzyme systems. This is important in the transmission of nerve impulses and contraction of muscles. It is essential for blood coagulation and present in the blood plasma in ionic form.

Symptoms of Calcium deficiency: Rickets in growing puppies, osteomalacia and osteoporosis in aged dogs, particularly in the multiparous bitches.

Other functions of Phosphorus: It is constituents of phosphoproteins, phospholipids and nucleic acids. It is actively involved in energy metabolism in the synthesis of sugar phosphates and the high energy phosphates (Adenosine triphosphate, ATP and adenosine diphosphate, ADP).

Symptoms of Phosphorus deficiency: Rickets in young and osteomalacia in mature dogs and daprived appetite (pica) in all age group are the common symptoms.

Magnesium: Like calcium and phosphorus, greater proportion of magnesium is utilized in bones and also, in muscles. It is a co-factor of many enzymes involved in important biochemical reactions in the body. Magnesium absorption from the intestine is affected by the dietary levels of calcium and phosphorus, and higher content of either in food decreases the availability of magnesium despite adequate supply in the diet.

Potassium, Sodium and Chloride: These ions alongwith bicarbonates are responsible for the maintenance of acid-base balance and osmotic regulation between the cellular and extracellular fluids. Foods are good sources of potassium, sodium and chloride are supplemented in the diets. Occurrence of deficiency is uncommon and can be observed only in dogs suffering from extended diarrhoea for several days accompanied with loss of appetite or vomiting.

The common symptoms of deficiency are generally non-specific like decreased food intake, poor growth, rough body coat, dehydration and weakness. The remedy is supplementation of a mixture of common salt, potassium chloride and sodium bicarbonate in the diets.

Iron: It is one of the most important trace element, essential for the formation of red blood corpuscles (RBC) and many enzymes mostly associated with the transportation of oxygen to cells and drawn of carbon dioxide from the cells for expulsion from the body in expired gases. Almost 90% of the 0.004 $ iron in the body is present in the form of haemoglobin, the coloured component of RBCs. The RBCs are replaced at a fast rate and life span is about 110 days in dogs. Recretion rate of iron is slow and the dogs receiving meat and fish rarely need additional iron supplementation but most of the dogs reared on strict vegetarian diets of Indian families receiving milk as source of animal protein may suffer from iron deficiency and require supplementation.

Iron deficiency or non-utilization of iron in the body causes anaemia due to defect in erythropoeisis. The anaemia is depicted by weakness, loss of body weight, retarded growth and flushed visible mucous membranes. Mother milk is deficient in iron despite dietary supplementation of its diet during lactation period due to barrier of passage of iron compound into the mammary glands. Thus, iron supplementation is required during the suckling period in puppies kept indoor in concrete house or cages fabricated of synthetic materials. Supply of copper and vitamin B_{12} is essential for the utilization of copper for haemoglobin formation in the blood cells. Excess dietary supply of iron compounds is also harmful and may cause phosphorus deficiency by interfering in the absorption of phosphorus due to formation of insoluble phosphate in the digestive tract.

Copper: The copper plays diversified roles in the body. It is required for the formation and maturation of erythrocytes, formation of collagen and elastic connective tissue, pig, entation of body coat and antioxident activities. The absorption rate of copper is very high (60-79%) in young growing puppies and gradually decreased to less than 20% in mature dogs. The copper is stored in liver, kidneys and brain. The availability of copper is reduced by dietary phytates, excess intake of vitamin C and high content of calcium, iron, molybdenum, zinc and sulphur and also, by heavy metals like lead, cadmium and silver, etc.

Deficiency of copper is rare in the dogs but some breeds often suffer from copper toxicity. Liver parenchyma of Doberman Pinscher, West Highland White Terrier and Bedlington Terrier has genetic affinity for copper, due to which in many dogs level becomes toxic. It may be better to get these breeds examined periodically for the copper toxicity.

Zinc: It plays important role in protein synthesis, conversion of carotenes into vitamin A activity, development of effective immune system and enzymes required for protection of cells from oxidation damage. The availability of zinc from complex with protein in natural foods is quite low. Phytates and fibres also reduce the availability of dietary zinc and it should be supplemented in the diets.

In some susceptible breeds, zinc deficiency occurs due to low absorption and it is manifested by the occurrence of dermatosis. The lesions are scaly skin around the snout, eyes, toes and foot pads. The condition is cured by treatment with zinc formulations administered under the supervision of a veterinary physician. Excess supplementation of zinc is also harmful and causes deficiency of copper and iron often leading to anaemia.

Manganese: It is a metal and present in traces in the tissues. The main organs containing higher amount of manganese than muscles are liver, kidneys, pancreas and bones. It is involved in metabolism of carbohydrates and protein as well as reproduction. It is an activator in many enzyme systems responsible for energy production, fatty acid synthesis and amino acid metabolism. It has compatibility with copper, zinc and iron, and may interchange in some of the enzyme systems.

Deficiency of manganese may cause retarted growth in young animals, deformity of bones and reproductive failure. Moreover, dogs are rarely affected by manganese deficiency. High content of calcium and phosphorus reduces its absorption from the intestine and may cause secondary deficiency.

Iodine: It is an essential constituent of thyroid hormones, triiodothyronine (T3) and thyroxine or tetraiodothyronine (T4) synthesized in the thyroid gland. The element is also present in the intermediate products monoidothyronine and diodothyronine in the process of T3 and T4 synthesis. These hormones regulate the basal energy metabolism in the body.

The thyroid gland attempts to compensate hormones supply in case of iodine deficiency. This causes hypertrophy of the gland which is known as goiter. The other symptoms of deficiency are retarded growth, alopesia and weakness. There may be abnormal increase in body mass.

Selenium: Earlier selenium was known for its toxicity but later on it was found to be an important trace element. It is a highly effective antioxident in conjunction with vitamin E. It is a component of enzyme glutathione peroxidase responsible for catalytic reaction for the removal of hydrogen peroxide, which damages cell membrane by oxidation. Food grains and meat are the good sources of selenium, and incidence of deficiency is rare.

Fluorine: It is required in very minute quantity for the normal growth of teeth and bones. Its deficiency may cause dental carries. It is also a very toxic element and its excess in diets may cause dental erosion, exposing even the pulp cavities on prolonged exposure. The other symptoms are exostosis of bones and joints deformities leading to lameness. It is not a problem in pet dogs. The toxicity may be observed in stray dogs of fluorine rich areas due to consumption of cadavers of ruminants.

6.12 Vitamins

The vitamins are highly variable nutrients without any considerable relationship in their chemical composition. These are required in minute amount and found in fat soluble and water soluble forms. The fat soluble vitamins are A, D, E and K; and water soluble vitamins are the members of B-complex and vitamin C.

i) Fat soluble vitamins

Vitamin A: It is present in the form of active vitamin A in the glands and other tissues of animals but in foods plant origin precursors of vitamin A, *i.e.* carotenes are present. The carotenes are converted into vitamin A activity in the intestinal epithelium and liver. All kinds of yellow grains, fruits and green vegetables are the good sources of carotenoids and liver, kidney and almost all fishes are the good sources of vitamin A. Normally deficiency of vitamin A are not encountered in dogs and if any, that may be due to other factors interfering in the utilization of carotenoids and vitamin A. Cat are not capable of converting carotenes into vitamin A activity to meet the requirements.

Vitamin D: The important active forms of vitamin D are: (1) the ergocalciferol or vitamin D2 and (2) the colecalciferol or vitamin D3. The later is a more stable compound due to higher tolerance of oxidation. Vitamin D acts like a hormone in the regulation of calcium metabolism in the body. Vitamin D participates in the absorption of calcium and phosphorus from the intestines and proper mineralization of the bones. It should be given in diets or should be provided adequate exposure to direct sunlight for the synthesis of vitamin. Thick body coat cover requires longer exposure to sunlight. Animal glands, flesh, fish, milk and egg yolk are the good sources of vitamin D.

Deficiency of vitamin D causes deformity of bones (rickets) in growing dogs due to incomplete and defective mineralization. Deformities may develop in foetii of bitches bearing large litter and receiving diets deficient or imbalanced in vitamin D alongwith the deficiency of calcium and phosphorus. Excess supplementation of vitamin D for long duration may be harmful due to hardening of soft tissues, particularly that of heart and kidneys.

Vitamin E: It is a cluster of identical active compounds. Eight natural forms of vitamin E are known. The most active form of vitamin E is alpha-tocopherol. The other forms are beta-, gama- and delta-tocopherols with side chain of saturated fatty acid. Another four compounds with side chain of unsaturated fatty acid possess little activity (less than 13% of alpha-tocopherol). This vitamin is stored in the body for a short time and should be supplied regularly in the diets. Green leaves, fruits and cereal grains are good sources of vitamin E but animal products are poor sources. Some of the activities of vitamin E can be accomplished by the traces of selenium but not all. Thus, vitamin E is an essntial dietary requirement.

Deficiency of vitamin E causes damage to cell wall in all kinds of tissues including the skin. It protects the cells from oxidative damage in conjunction with selenium and cysteine. Occurrence of deficiency is not known on normal feeding.

Vitamin K: This vitamin is present in different chemical forms in the vegetables, egg yolk, liver and fish adequate to meet the requirements. A small quantity is also produced by the common enteric bacteria. Vitamin K1 present in plants is called phylloquinone and that of microbial origin is the menaquinone. It is a clotting agent present in the blood. The requirement of vitamin K is quite less and chance of deficiency is remote.

ii) Water soluble vitamins

These are vitamins of B-complex group and vitamin C (Ascorbic acid). These vitamins are not stored in the body and most of them should be available in the diets. The members of vitamin B-complex group are the co-enzyme in different enzyme systems of metabolism. Vitamin B-complex includes thiamine, riboflavin, niacin, pyridoxne, biotin, pantothenic acid, folic acid, choline and cyanocobalamine (vitamin B_{12}).

Vitamin C (Ascorbic acid)

This vitamin is required for the synthesis of collagen. Dogs and cats do not require this vitamin.

6.13 Processing of Foods

Since environmental pollution is increasing and spreading every day, it will not be wise to advise the feeding of raw foods other than fruits. The different methods used for the processing of dog's food are cooking, boiling, steaming, roasting, toasting, shredding and extruding, etc. Processing of foods is done for increasing the voluntary intake of food by improving palatability and increasing the digestibility of foods and absorption of nutrients. Commercial dog foods are dispensed in dry form, semi-solid form and canned moist foods.

Effects of cooking on food: Some significant changes occur due to cooking in the physical form and sometimes in chemical composition of foods. These changes are mostly helpful in the better digestion of foods and utilization of nutrients in the body. The various changes in foods due to cooking are:

1. An increase in the volume provides larger area for the action of digestive enzymes and thereby increases digestion.
2. Rupture of cells of foods releases nutritional constituents for digestion.
3. Denaturation of proteins. In this process, some harmful constituents like trypsin inhibitors are destroyed. It also helps in enzymic digestion.
4. Gelatinization of starch helps in effective enzymic digestion.
5. Almost all infectious organisms are killed in the Indian system of cooking.
6. Use of flavouring agents (spices and condiments) works as appetizers and increases the secretion of saliva.
7. However, there is considerable loss of eat labile vitamins, particularly vitamin B-complex and vitamin C.
8. Cooking on direct fire also causes loss of some nutrients.

Methods of cooking: One or more of the following methods are used for cooking foods:

1. Traditional Indian system of cooking using pans, tawa, bhagona, etc.
2. Cooking on direct fire , *viz.* roasting, toasting, etc.
3. Pressure cooking.
4. Cooking in hot air oven.
5. Cooking in microwave oven.

Palatability score of diets: Table 1 has been suggested for determining the relative voluntary intake of foods and diets.

Table 1. Determination of palatability score in dogs.

Score	Response of dogs during trial
1	High palatability is indicated by voluntary intake of optimum quantity without hesitation and reluctance.
2	Less attention on food but voluntary intake is optimum in longer duration.
3	Refuses to eat after eating a portion and prefer to remain hungry.
4	Dogs initially smell the food or diet for testing and then turn away despite offering for longer duration (30 to 60 minutes).

6.14 Functional Foods

It is a recent terminology for characterizing the foods probably used first time by the Japanese nutritionists for the foods that supply ingredients, in addition to normal nutrients, that meet the requirements of specific functions in the body. At present, the definitions of functional foods in vogue are:

1. The functional foods provide a health benefit beyond the traditional nutrients present in such foods (Institute of Medicine's Food and Nutrition Board).
2. The foods that provide health benefits beyond basic nutrients are the functional foods (International Food Information Council, IFIC).

The functional foods are used for increasing specific physiological functions for the prevention and cure of some diseases. It appears difficult to draw a line between the functional foods and the protective foods like Chyawanprash and Linseed laddoo used in human diets since thousands of years.

Methods of obtaining functional foods: Following methods may be used for obtaining the functional foods:

1. Addition of some components in the foods from the other sources.
2. Removal of some constituents from the original foods.
3. Modification of composition of foods by food processing technologies.

4. Modification of physical and chemical forms of foods by treatments. This may be physical, chemical or biological treatment either alone or combined.

Types of functional foods: The functional foods have been differentiated into prebiotics, probiotics and symbiotics. Last one is the combination of first two types.

i) Prebiotics

These are food ingredients that remain largely undigested in the small intestine. These constituents of foods impart beneficial effects by: (a) selective stimulation of growth of normal microflora in the intestine and (b) also stimulating the functions of these bacteria. The action is more specific in colon and helpful in improving the health of colon.

Different sources of prebiotics: Some of the common prebiotics are starches, fibre in foods, sugar alcohol. Other oligosaccharides are the fructo-oligosaccharides (FOS), insulin, fructans and iso-malto oligosaccharides (lactilol, lactosucrose, lactulose and pyrodextrins), transgalacto-oligosaccharides, xylo-oligo-saccharides and mannon-oligosaccharides.

Natural sources of prebiotics: These are Soya-oligosaccharides (trisaccharide raffinose and tetrasaccaride stachyose), and Chicory insulin, fructan.

Non-digestible insulin like fructans are present in vegetables, fruits and food grains.

The oligosaccharides are the glycosides of less than 10 molecules of hexose or pentose units.

The commercial synthetic prebiotics are inulins and oligofructose.

Prebiotic has been also defined as a selectively fermented ingredient of food that allows specific changes in the composition as well as activities in the microbial inhabitants of the alimentary canal that confers benefits upon the host welfare and health.

Some of the important action of prebiotic chicory (Cichorium intybus) also known as kasani, succory and hinduba are presented in Table 2.

Table 2. Effect of prebiotics on some physiological functions of the gut and their therapeutic actions.

Action of physiological functions of gut	Therapeutic role
1. Composition and action of gut microbial by population is favourably changed.	Improvement of enteric health inactivating or destroying pathogens.
2. Improvement in consistency of faeces and defecation.	Improvent in irritable diseases of the intestines.
3. Improvement in absorption of minerals through the healthy intestinal wall.	Prevention of rickets in young ones and osteoporosis in aged ones.
4. Production of endocrine peptides.	Protection from colon cancer.
5. Improvement in immunity and resistence.	Protection from many infections.
6. Maintenance of lipids and glucose.	Protection from obesity and diabetes mellitus.

ii) Probiotics

Generally following three definitions are used for describing the probiotics:

1. Probiotics are the organisms and substances that influence the intestinal microflora balance in animals (R B Parker, 1974).
2. Probiotic is a live microbial feed additive, which benefit the host animal by improving its intestinal microbial balance (R Fuller, 1989).
3. Probiotic is a live microbial feed supplement that is beneficial to health (S Salminen, A C Ouweliand and E Isolauri, 1998).

The three definitions are more or less similar and can be summarized as, "The probiotic is a live micro-organism capable of imparting beneficial effects for the host either by balancing the normal microbial population in the intestines or by liberating substances for the elimination and destruction of harmful microorganisms".

Characteristics of an ideal Probiotic

1. It should be preferably one or more member of normal microbes inhabiting the intestine of host animal.

2. It must be non-pathogenic capable of thriving and multiplying in the almost anaerobic environment of intestines.
3. It should be capable to bear the stress of processing.
4. It should not be destroyed by gastric acid and bile during passage to intestines.
5. The probiotics should be safe for handling during preparation and consumption.
6. It adheres to intestinal epithelium and mucous.
7. It persists and grow in the intestinal environment.
8. Synthesizes compounds for the inhibition of harmful micro-organisms.
9. Probiotic works as modulation factor in development of immune system.
10. It is associated with cholesterol assimilation, lactase activity and vitamin production.

Various microbial probiotics: These may be members of one or more groups. Major group of probiotics belong to lactic acid bacteria (LAB). Important microbial species and their strains to be used as probiotic are presented in Table 3.

Table 3. Species and strains of micro-organisms used as probiotic.

Species/ group/class	Strains
Lactobacilli	Lactobacillus acidophilus, L. casei, L.rhaminosus, L. reuteri, L. plantarum, L. gasseri ADH, L. johnsoni LA1, L. delbrueckii, L. brevis, L. bulgaricus, L. fermentum, L. halveticus, L. curvatus and L.cellobiosus.
Bifidobacterium	B. bifidum, B. breve, B. infantus, B. adolescentis, B. animalis, B. longum, B. thermophilum.
Gram positive cocci	Enterococcus faecium, Streptococcus thermophilus and Lactococcus lactis.
Yeast	Saccharomyces cerevisiae and S. boulardii.
Fungi	Aspergillus orizae and Scitolidium acidophilus.

Mode of action of probiotics

Although exact action of probiotics is not yet fully known, indeed some mode of action has been speculated:

1. Chemical inhibition of harmful enteric micro-organisms.
2. Stimulation of beneficial micro-organisms in the intestines.
3. Competition for nutrients.
4. Stimulation of immunogenic system.
5. Higher affinity for adhesion receptors.
6. Production of bacteriocins having antagonistic action against closely related to producer bacteria.
7. Modulation of the function of intestinal microbial inhabitants.
8. Barrier effect for protection against pathogenic micro-organisms.
9. Trophic functions of probiotics control the immune homeostasis of the gut.
10. Prevention of multiplication and pathogenic action of the disease causing micro-organisms invading the gut.
11. Synthesis of volatile fatty acids (VFAs) and lactic acid lowers the pH of gut and prevents the detrimental action of pathogenic micro-organisms.

Beneficial effects of probiotics

1. Reduction and as far as possible elimination of the disease producing micro-organisms and their toxins from the alimentary tract of the host.
2. Release of nutrients, antioxidants, growth factors and coagulation factors.
3. Regularization of normal gut motility.
4. Modulation of innate and adaptive immune defense mechanism through the normalization of disturbed gut microbiota.
5. Reduction in the level of blood cholesterol and other unwanted lipids.
6. Significant increase in erythrocytes, haematocrit, haemoglobin, leucocytes (neutrophils, monocytes), serum immunoglobulins and

reduction in erythrocyte fragility and serum nitrous oxide concentration due to feeding of Lactobacillus acidophilus.

7. Increase in serum proteins and total lipids and reduction in serum glucose level.

iii) Symbiotics

These are mixtures of selected prebiotics and probiotics of synergistic nature. These are colonic food with probiotic and prebiotic properties of functional food used for health improvement.

Beneficial effects of symbiotics

1. Active repair of damaged gut mucosa.
2. Inhibition of the pathogenic micro-organisms.
3. Rehabilitation of the normal microbiota of the gut.
4. Establishment of useful micro-organisms in the gut.
5. Improvement of immune system.
6. Prevention of enteric cancer.
7. Reduction of serum tryglycerides, cholesterol and foul smell emitting compounds like ammonia, skatole, indole, p-cresol and phenols.

6.15 Nutrients Requirement of Domestic Dogs

The nutritional requirements suggested by the National Research Council (NRC) of the National Academy of Sciences and another suggested by the Association of American Feed Control Official (AAFCO) are more commonly used for the manufacture of commercial foods of dogs and also, for the feeding of dog breeding kennels. In recent years, commercial manufacture of dry and moist foods of dogs has shown a rising trend due to increase in urbanization coupled with dog keeping. Families of working couple in cities mostly living with or without parent (generally retired and aged) and one or two children though keep a dog of small or medium size breed but only in few cases try to have basic informations about the food requirements and feeding behaviour. Such families are dependent on commercial ready to feed processed foods marketed either in the form of a calculated diet for different body weights and physiological state or in the form of dry bulk packaging for feeding according to instruction supplied by the food manufacturing company.

The nutrient requirements of growing pups as per NRC, 1985) and AAFCO (1998) are presented in Table 4.

Table 4. Nutrients requirement of growing pups (per kg body weight per day).

		As per NRC (1985)		As per AAFCO (1998)	
Nutrients		**Unit**	**Amount**	**Unit**	**Amount**
A	ENERGY			kcal per g	3.5
B	FAT	g	2.70	%	8.0
	Linoleic acid	g	0.54	%	1.0
C	PROTEIN			%	22.00
	Essential Amino acids				
	Arginine	mg	274	%	0.62
	Histidine	,,	98	,,	0.22
	Isoleucine	,,	196	,,	0.45
	Leucine	,,	318	,,	0.72
	Lysine	,,	280	,,	0.77
	Methionine + cystine	,,	212	,,	0.53
	Phenylalanine + Tyrosine		390	,,	0.89
	Threonine	,,	254	,,	0.58
	Tryptophan	,,	82	,,	0.20
	Valine	,,	210	,,	0.48
	Dispensible amino acids	,,	3414		
D	MINERALS				
	Calcium	,,	320	,,	1.00
	Phosphorus	,,	240	,,	0.80
	Potassium	,,	240	,,	0.60
	Sodium	,,	30	,,	0.30
	Chloride	,,	46	,,	0.45
	Magnesium	,,	22	,,	0.04
	Iron	,,	1.74	,,	80.00
	Copper	,,	0.16	,,	7.30

	Manganese	,,	0.28	,,	5.00
	Zinc	,,	1.94	,,	120.00
	Iodine	,,	0.03	,,	1.50
	Selenium	ug	6.00	,,	0.11
E	VITAMINS				
	Vitamin A	IU	202.00	IU/kg	5000.00
	Vitamin D	,,	22.00	,,	500.00
	Vitamin E	,,	1.20	,,	50.00
	Thiamine	ug	54.00	mg/kg	10.000
	Riboflavin	,,	100.00	,,	2.200
	Pantothenic acid	,,	400.00	,,	1.000
	Pyridoxine	,,	60.00	,,	1.000
	Niacin	,,	450.00	,,	11.400
	Folic acid	,,	8.00	,,	0.180
	Vitamin B12	,,	1.00	,,	0.022
	Choline	mg	50.00	,,	1200.000

NB: NRC (per kg body weight per day) and AAFCO (in food on Dry matter basis)

The minimum nutrients content in the composite foods of dogs suggested by AAFCO (1998) is presented in Table 5.

Table 5. Minimum Nutrients content in foods containing 3500 kcal ME per kg on dry matter basis.

Nutrients	Growth & Reproduction	Maintenance of Adults
Protein	22 %	18 %
Essential Amino Acids (% in food)		
Arginine	0.62	0.51
Histidine	0.22	0.18
Isoleucine	0.45	0.37
Leucine	0.72	0.59
Lysine	0.77	0.63
Methionine + cystine	0.53	0.43
Phenylalanine + tyrosine	0.89	0.73

Threonine	0.58	0.48
Tryptophan	0.20	0.16
Valine	0.48	0.39
Fat		
Linoleic acid	1.00	1.00
Minerals		
Calcium	1.00	0.60 (upto 2.5)
Phosphorus	0.80	0.50 (upto 1.6)
Ca : P ratio	1 : 1	1 : 1 (2 : 1)
Potassium	0.60	0.60
Sodium	0.30	0.06
Chloride	0.45	0.09
Magnesium	0.04	0.04 (upto 0.3)
Iron (mg/ kg food)	80	80 (upto 3000)
Copper	7.3	7.3
Manganese	5.0	5.0
Zinc	120	120 (upto 1000)
Iodine	1.50	1.50 (upto 50)
Selenium	0.11	0.11
Vitamins		
Vitamin A (IU/kg)	5000	5000 (upto 25000)
Vitamin D (IU/kg)	500	500 (upto 5000)
Vitamin E (IU/kg)	50	50 (upto 1000)
Water soluble vitamins (mg/kg)		
Thiamine	1.0	1.0
Riboflavin	2.2	2.2
Pantothenic acid	10.0	10.0
Niacin	11.4	11.4
Pyridoxine	1.0	1.0
Folic acid	0.18	0.18
Vitamin B12	0.022	0.022
Choline	1200	1200
ME (kcal/kg food dry matter)	3500	3500

i) Nutritional Composition of Diets as per SSNIFT

The requirements given on the basis of proximate principles will be more convenient for use at places lacking facilities of expensive instruments. Nutrients requirement for maintenance and breeding are presented in Table 6.

Table 6. Nutritional composition of diets for maintenance and breeding

Nutrients	Maintenance food	Breeding dogs diet
Metabolizable Energy	12 Mj per kg food	13.5 Mj per kg food
Crude Protein (CP%)	22.0	25.0
Ether Extract (EE%)	5.5	7.5
Crude Fibre (CF%)	4.8	4.8
Total Ash %	7.2	7.0
Minerals (%)		
Calcium (Ca)	1.20	1.20
Phosphorus (P)	1.00	1.00
Magnesium (Mg)	0.22	0.22
Sodium (Na)	0.44	0.44
Potassium (K)	0.00	1.00
Amino Acids (%)		
Arginine	1.50	1.70
Cysteine	0.40	0.35
Glycine	1.40	1.40
Histidine	0.60	0.60
Isoleucine	0.90	1.00
Leucine	1.70	1.00
Lysine	1.50	1.70
Methionine	0.60	0.60
Phenylalanine	1.00	1.20
Tryptophan	0.30	0.30
Valine	1.10	1.30
Trace minerals 'per kg food'		
Manganese (Mn, mg)	50	50
Copper (Cu, mg)	12	12
Zinc (Zn, mg)	60	60
Iodine (I, mg)	1	1.4
Iron (Fe, mg)	250	300
Fluorine (F, mg)	<25	<15

Vitamins supplement for both (per kg of food)

Vitamin A	17000 IU
Vitamin D3	1000 IU
Vitamin E	200 mg
Vitamins B1, B2 and B6	15 mg each
Vitamin B12	50 ug
Biotin	500 ug
Pantothenic acid	12 mg
Choline	1500 mg
Nicotinic acid (Niacin)	25 mg
Folic acid	4 mg
Inositol	200 mg

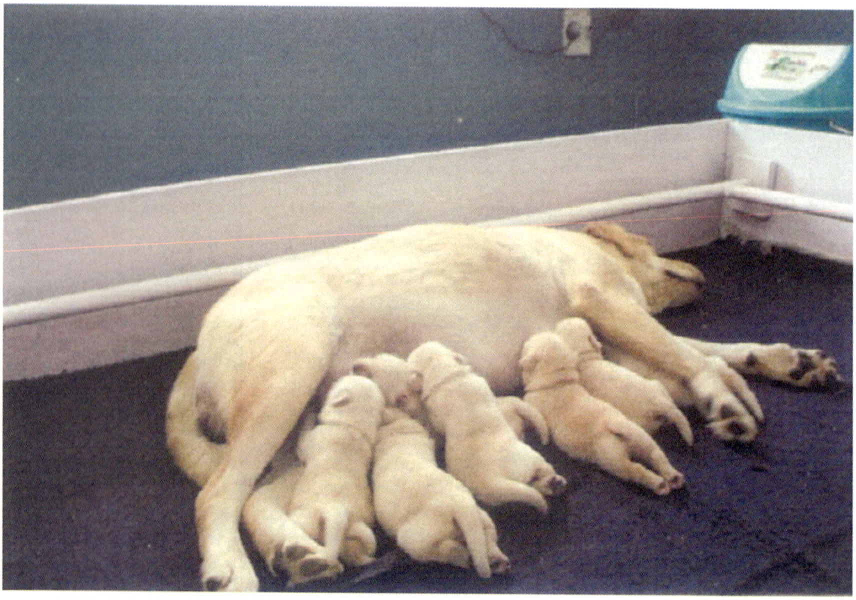

Fig. 6.1 Labrador Retriever bitch and litter

❑❑❑

Chapter 7

Dietary Management of Sick Dog

Special diets are often required for the feeding of sick dogs suffering from different kinds of systemic disorders and other diseases, particularly in the clinico-pathological disturbances of the gastrointestinal tract, heart problems, renal problems, osteal disorders and cutaneous problems, etc.

7.1 Points Requiring Attention

1. For symptomatic treatments, easily digestible foods are used for the preparation of therapeutic diets.
2. Specific dietary therapy is quite difficult and requires thorough veterinary skill and characteristic of different kinds of foods for correct selection of ingredients.
3. The therapeutic diets are formulated by eliminating reactive foods. It means the preparation of as far as possible the non-allergic diets.
4. In some kinds of disorders, low fat diets containing medium chain triglycerides (MCT) are required. For this purpose, use of oil may be needed.
5. In some other kind of diseases, low energy fibrous diet is required.
6. In deficiency diseases, different kinds of corrective formulations are required.
7. In few diseases, elimination of one or more sources of nutrients (natural foods or synthetic supplements) may be necessary.

7.2 Therapeutic Nutrition

The use of specific nutrient(s) for the cure of an ailment or enhancing the cure by supportive action is therapeutic nutrition.

7.3 Therapeutic Diets

The special diets prepared from the specific food ingredient for the supply of determined level of nutrients are the therapeutic diets.

7.4 Veterinary Nutrition

The therapeutic nutrition applied to animals is known as veterinary nutrition.

i) Veterinary Dietetics

The application of fundamental nutrition and veterinary nutrition for the formulation of special diets for ailing animals is known as veterinary dietetics. It also includes the technology of preparation and methods of feeding.

7.5 Blend Diets or Easily Digestible Diets

Such diets are used for the feeding of patients suffering from inflammatory conditions of the digestive system like gastritis, enteritis, gastroenteritis and colitis, etc. The foods used for the preparation of blend diets are commonly found in most of the homes and also, available in the local markets. The common foods used for the formulation of blend diets are paneer, cottage cheese, chhenna, tender green beans, rice, potatoes, sweet potato, carrot, low fat chicken or flesh of young animals (veal, lamb, etc). The diets are prepared by boiling meat or milk products with rice or potato in 1:2 ratio approximately. These diets are low in lactose except the diets with skim milk, low in fat and easily digestible. In the patients with lactose intolerance use of milk in the diets should be prohibited. These diets are fed in small amount at short intervals to avoid the undesired loading of stomach. This is continued until patient shows the signs of recovery from the diarrhoea, dysentery or indigestion, etc. This is followed by gradual shifting of convalescing patient on normal diet feds fed before earlier in healthy condition. Feeding of balanced blend diets may be continued for some time even after recovery in case of young animals and very old dogs.

The blend diets have been found to be useful for reducing and preventing the emesis (vomiting). These diets are normally made of non-sugar carbohydrates (starch rich foods) and contain small amount of fat and fibre. Use of excess salt and minerals should be avoided in the preparation of blend diets because these are hyper osmolar and may delay the normal evacuation of gastric compartments. Such diets may also delay gastro-intestinal clearance, as the dogs are unable to digest sugars due to lack of sucrase enzyme production in the digestive system.

7.6 Elimination Diets

These diets are composed for the replacement of the diets currently fed to the animals and suspected to be responsible for the delay in recovery or synergistic in action or even the cause of ailment. The elimination diets are prepared from the simple and highly digestible ingredients supplemented with essential minerals and vitamins. The efficacy assessment of such diets takes about 3-4 weeks of feeding trial and in some cases, trial duration may be even longer (6-8 weeks). During the entire period of feeding trial, the feeding of any other food even casually is not permitted. After establishing the efficacy of elimination diet of a fully defined recipe, the recovered animal may be gradually reverted back to feeding of common wholesome foods used for feeding before the sickness.

7.7 Fibre Rich Diets

Dietary fibre is the less digestible or so called indigestible fraction of the foods used for the composition of suitably balanced diets. In the proximate analysis system, this fraction is called crude fibre and in the detergent system of analysis, it is separated as two types, i.e. neutral detergent fibre (NDF) and acid detergent fibre (ADF). Some clinicians use the term soluble and insoluble dietary fibre but such strict fibre fractions are not present in the natural foods. High fibre diets are required for the management of different kinds of gastrointestinal disorders due to disturbances of physiological functions or due to occurrence of clinico-pathological changes. Use of high fibre diets is more advantageous in the management of enteric disorders specially the digestive disorders of the large intestine.

The characteristics of dietary fibre may be changed significantly with the use of different processing methods. Soaking in water, cooking and grinding increases the rate of microbial digestion of fibrous fraction of the diets. This happens due to increase in the area of action or due to softening of the foods. Large proportion of residual undigested fibre increases the volume of faeces that stimulates easy defecation. Some amount of insoluble fraction in the digesta probably helps in the correction of myoelectrical activity of the colon and helps to prevent the spasmodic contractions. Short chain volatile fatty acids (VFA) are produced in the large intestine from the microbial fermentation of the cellulose and hemicellulose components of the dietary fibre fraction. The VFAs are absorbed in the body pool and utilized for the supply of energy. However, energy supply from the dietary fibre fraction is very less in the dogs.

Non-inflammatory and to some extent, mild inflammatory diarrhoea due to disorders of the large intestine is often corrected by increasing the dietary level of fibre fraction. This also helps in relieving the constipation by physical action of increasing the rate of passage of digesta through exerting pressure on the wall of the intestine. Although animals suffering from non-inflammatory constipation responds in few days but feeding of such diets may be continued for 2-3 weeks. Coarse wheat bran is one of the suitable and rasily available source of dietary fibre for the therapeutic purpose.

7.8 Low Allergenic and Non-Allergenic Diets

Allergenic reaction of some foods and food constituents is often encountered in the domesticated dogs. This may be either: (i) non-immune mediated or (ii) immune mediated reactions. In such cases, history of the food ingredients used for the preparation of diet fed to the suffering animals during the immediate past few days is traced and examined for the presence of allergenic factors, which may be a protein, amino acid, pigment or some non-nutritional constituent. Such foods are immediately replaced from the diet of the reacting dogs, if identified; otherwise entire diet is replaced with a diet of non-allergenic food ingredients. This is not an easy task and hit and trial method is time consuming. For all practical purpose, low allergenic diets and elimination diets may be reasonably useful. A few examples of such diets are as follows:

1. Skin and adipose tissue removed chicken, duck, goose, turkey or pigeon meat 30%, boiled and pilled potato (smashed) 70%. This is a satisfactory low allergenic diet.
2. Bones and spicules removed boiled white fish 35% and boiled, pilled and smashed potato 65%.

From these two diets, meat and fish may be replaced with paneer or chakka on equal protein basis, and potato can be replaced with noiled polished rice. There may be need of supplementing low density lipids (unsaturated fatty acids rich edible oils), minerals and vitamins for balancing the diets, when feeding period is likely to extend beyond two weeks.

7.9 Liquid Diets (Fluid Therapy)

The administration of nutritional fluid preparations like isotonic saline, isotonic dextrose saline and easily metabolizable nutritional fluid preparations is required either in emergency for the restoration of body fluid level as in the case of dehydration or the administration of nutrients mixture, when animal is unable to eat or drink or refuse to eat and drink. The various clinico-pthological conditions requiring the use of fluid therapy are dehydration, disturbance in the concentration of electrolytes and disturbance of acid-base status of the body fluid compartments, and shock due to the physical or chemical causes. In the dogs, severe vomiting (expulsion of mostly gastric but sometimes intestinal contents also) causes the occurrence of hypokalamic condition. The hypokalamia may or may not be associated with acidosis. The other conditions causing hypokalamia are the anuric renal failure and hypoadrenocorticism. Clinical symptoms are not sufficient to help the correct prediction in the nature of electrolytes and acid-base changes in the body fluids. Therefore, it is necessary to determine the concentration of electrolytes in the serum. However, normal saline alongwith a dilute solution of potassium chloride at the rate of 20 meq per litre may be administered. For the correct supplementation of potassium in fluid therapy, the following guidelines should be followed, i.e. for the serum potassium concentration of more than 3.5, 3.0-3.5, 2.5-3.0, 2.0-2.5 and less than 2.0 meq per litre of serum, potassium supplement per litre of physiological fluid may be kept around 20, 30, 40, 60 and 80 meq, respectively. Administration of therapeutic fluid should be limited to maintain total supply of not more than 0.5 meq per kg body weight per hour.The fluid administration is either equivalent to maintenance requirement or double the requirement and the dose is determined on the basis of the condition and severity of the ailment.

There may be need of bicarbonate administration in very rare cases and should be used carefully because its administration may cause acidosis. Therefore, it should not be mixed with the normal saline.

i) Body conditions requiring parentral fluid therapy

The following conditions of body determine the need of parentral administration of therapeutic fluids or liquid diets:

1. In the animals suffering from shock.
2. In cases of severe diarrhoea and dysentery causing dehydration.
3. Obstruction in the gastrointestinal tract.
4. Inflammation of the gastrointestinal tract inhibiting the absorption of fluid and nutrients into the body compartments.
5. Frequent vomiting particularly shortly after the oral administration of the therapeutic fluid or other foods and water.

Normally therapeutic fluids should be administered through intravenous (IV) route and for this purpose a canula may be placed IV at a suitable place on the body for the duration of therapy. Jugular vein is considered a suitable site and free end of canula is secured by retention suture. The canula is kept petent by filling dilute solution of anticoagulent like heparin. In some rare cases, intramedullary route can be used. Intra-peritoneal route may be also used but its use is very risky, as little laxity in hygiene may cause peritonitis.

7.10 Diseases requiring Fluid Therapy

1. Shock exhibited by tachycardia.
2. Weak peripheral perfusion.
3. Extremities are weak.
4. Capillary refill requires much longer time.
5. Pulse is weak.
6. In case of tachypnoea.

Dose of therapeutic fluid: This depends on the condition of body and the disease. The dose ranges from 80 to 90 ml per kg body weight but in some emergency, it may be increased to 100 ml per kg body weight. Preferred route for the administration of fluid is the jugular vein. Ringer's solution may contain lsctate and it should be administered very slowly by intravenous route. Alternate of normal saline is the use of hypertonic saline solution. This solution is used to reduce the administration of large volume of fluid in the patients of shock. However, intravenous administration of hypertonic saline is a highly skilled job. A 7% saline solution is administered at the rate of 4-5 ml per kg body weight in about 10-12 minutes. Infusion of total hypertonic saline should not exceed 10 ml per kg body weight. Use of a mixture of 7% saline and 7% glucose has been found to be more effective for the treatment of shock, and it can also be administered at a relatively faster rate of 3-5 ml per kg body weight in about 5-6 minutes time; and it is limited to maximum 10 ml per kg body weight. Administration of hypertonic solutions should be discontinued after reaching the level of 160 meq per litre of serum. Administration of normal saline may be continued, if necessary, but its rate should be limited to 10-20 ml per kg body weight per hour to control the shock. Colloids are also useful for the treatment of shock and the mechanism is similar to that of hypertonic solution.

Administration of hypertonic fluid for the therapeutic uses are contraindicated in the following systemic disorders:

1. The hypernatremic dehydration.
2. The cordiogenic shock.
3. The renal failure and
4. The uncontrolled haemorrhage.

For the correction of dehydration, administration of equivalent volume of physiological solution is required. For this purpose, the degree of dehydration is assessed on the basis of the following changes in the body texture of the patient:

1. The colour of skin turns darker at 5-6% dehydration, and the skin tainting is coupled with loss in body weight in almost all the patients. Moreover, sign of skin tainting generally does not appear in obese animals and per acute or sudden dehydration.
2. The oral mucuous membrane becomes dry and rough at about 6-7% dehydration in the dogs. These changes should be differentiated with the help of other changes because moist oral mucuous membrane is seen in dehydrated dogs showing nausea. On the other hand, it may be dry in hydrated dogs suffering from some of the respiratory disorders like panting and dyspnoea.

The level of dehydration is multiplied with the body weight of the dehydrated dog in kilogram for estimating the requirement of the physiological fluid for administration for the restoration of body fluid volume.The estimated volume of therapeutic fluid should be administered through intravenous route in 2 to 8 hours period depending on the condition and response of the patient. It is advised to infuse about 10% more fluid than the estimated requirement. However, much excess administration of fluid may be harmful in the animals suffering from the following ailments:

1. Congenital heart failure.
2. Oligouric renal failure.
3. Anuric renal failure.
4. Pulmonary oedema.
5. Anaemia and.
6. Ecterus or jaundice.

Therapeutic fluid may be also administered by sub-cutaneous (SC) route and can be easily repeated for several times-if the needle and syringe are sterilized properly, else disposable syringe and needle should be used. About 10 to 50 ml of the therapeutic fluid may be deposited at several place beneath the skin depending on the need of fluid and size of the patient. However, diffusion of fluid from the dependent parts of the body is very slow. The sub-cutaneous (SC) route of fluid infusion is not suitable in the case of severe dehydration, but it can be used after the initial intravenous administration.

For the maintenance of fluid compartments, sub-cutaneous (SC) route may be more convenient and for this purpose about 50 to 60 ml physiological fluid per kg body weight is required daily. A higher level of more than 60 ml per kg body weight daily is used for the small breeds while 5 ml per kg body weight is used for the medium and large breeds. Selection of appropriate therapeutic fluid is important for the maintenance of electrolytes balance. The systemic disorders causing excessive vomiting, diarrhoea and urination cause continued loss of body weight due to dehydration and loss in body weight may be used for the approximate assessment of therapeutic fluid requirement. For the use of fluid therapy, a suitable method should be selected for the estimation of fluid requirement. Insufficient fluid infusion results in progressive loss of body weight.

Over hydration is also harmful and may be responsible for the development of other disorders like :

1. Inspiratory pulmonary crackles.
2. Systolic cardiac murmur and
3. Oedema (gallop rhythm) of the neck region.

7.11 Rehydration Therapy

It is possible in patients drinking fluid and for this purpose glucose, fructose or amino acids are mixed with the normal saline. This therapy can be used only when there is no emesis and the intestines are healthy and functional for the absorption and transportation of the therapeutic fluid.

i) Therapeutic fluid requirement for the correction of Hypoproteinimia

The level of hypoalbumenia determines the composition of therapeutic fluid and its quantity for administration. Infusion of normal saline or glucose (dextrose) saline may further complicate the problem by further reducing the level of serum albumin and associated function, osmotic pressure. This may result in the occurrence of ascites, extensive oedema and peripheral perfusion. Severe hypoalbuminemia due to drop of serum albumin level below 1.5g per 100 ml may require blood or plasma transfusion.

7.12 Special Supplemental Feeding

In the severe cases of nutritional deficiency, caused by various degree of decrease in food intake, decreased digestibility or decrease in absorption or availability of the nutrient (s), use of special nutritional supplementation is required. The need of nutritional supplementation of the animals depends on the following factors:

1. Breed of the dog.
2. Age of the dog.
3. Physiological state of the body, viz. growth, pregnancy, lactation and old age.
4. Climatic conditions specially the ambient temperature and humidity.
5. Clinical condition or soundness of the dog.

Energy and protein are considered first among all the nutrients required for the maintenance of optimum physiological functions. The maintenance requirement of energy and protein vary to some extent in the sick animals particularly in the cases of traumatic and inflammatory conditions as shown in Table 1.

Table 1. Estimation of the energy and protein requirement for maintenance of dogs.

Details	Values
Basal energy requirement	30 X W (kg) + 70 kcal/ day
For dogs below 2 kg and more than 25 kg, the values of metabolic body weight ($W^{0.75}$) is used as,	70 X $W^{0.75}$ kcal/day
ME requirement of dogs for maintenance (kcal/day),	BMR x adjustment factor
For dogs resting in confinement	1.25
During convulscence after surgery	1.30
After traumatic injury	1.50
For patients of sepsis	1.70
For patients of severe burns	2.00
Protein requirement of adult dogs per day	4 g/kg body weight

Average value of ME requirement for the maintenance of adult dogs is 70 kcal per kg body weight, which is equivalent to 125 kcal per kg $W^{0.75}$.

i) Tube feeding

It is a skilled job of feeding the liquid diet containing easily flowing nutrients (foods or synthetic diet or therapeutic fluid) in the form of solution, suspension and fine particles. Various methods used for tube feeding are listed as follows:

1. Orally inserted tube in the oesophagus or upto cordia in stomach.
2. Nasopharyngeal inserted feeding tube.
3. Use of pharyngostomy tube.
4. Use of oesophagotomy tube.
5. Use of gastrotomy tube.
6. Use of enterostomy tube.

ii) Parentral feeding

Parentral feeding becomes necessary, when imgestion of food or absorption of nutrients fails to provide nutritional requirements from the infested foods. It is required in the extensive inflammatory condition of the alimentary canal, diarrhoea and dysentery. The management of catheter in the jugular vein is very risky and in hot and humid-hot climatic conditions of the tropical countries, it is rather more difficult to maintain aseptic condition for several days except in very few well-equipped veterinary hospitals.

7.13 Grass Eating by Dogs

Occassional grass eating instinct in dogs is quite common and generally, it indicates gastro-intestinal disturbances or some kind of error in the diets of the dogs. In most of the cases, dogs eat green grass to facilitate the expulsion of worms from the digestive tract. The irritation caused by the worms or any other factors in the alimentary tract, constipation due to eating of low fibre diets and other gastric disorders stimulates the dogs to eat grass. The dogs kept under strict confinement are not exposed to grass eating and in lieu they eat rugs, bedding material, hairs or skin of the small animals which they kill the game. Some dogs eat a small amount of green grass, when their diets do not contain fruits and vegetables for several days.

In the clinico-pathological conditions, the grass eating is mostly followed by vomiting. One should not panic from grass eating of his pet dog unless it becomes habit and does not stop after one or two vomitings in a few hours time. Sometimes grass eating may not be associated with any kind of gastro-enteric problem and almost 90 per cent dogs eat grass at one or the other time, and it has no relationship with the age, sex and size of the dog.

7.14 Feeding of Bones to Dogs

The mouth specially the jaws and teeth of the dogs have been evolved for catching, holding and tearing the game or carcass and chewing the bones after eating the flesh. Thus, the mouth is made for hard work during eating the prey in wild dogs, and food in domesticated dogs as evident from the well-developed and distinctly strong canine teeth. The digestive system of dog has also evolved for digesting flesh, adipose tissue and bones. Therefore, the physical form of foods should be both soft as well as hard for adequate working of the jaws and teeth during eating. For the maintenance of teeth and gums in good health, the pet dogs kept in confinement should be offered healthy fresh or partially boiled long bones. In the strict vegetarian households as in many Indian families, the bones may be replaced with hard biscuits and artificial bone-shaped hard objects should be provided for chewing. Chewing of bones does not allow the deposition of tartar on the teeth which is responsible for providing multiplication places for the micro-organisms causing occurrence of gum sores resulting in weakening of the teeth, pyorrhea and loosening and falling of the teeth.

Chewing of bones also supplies adequate amount of various essential minerals specially the calcium, phosphorus, magnesium and iron present abundantly in the bones and bone marrow. It also provides lipids and proteins from the marrow. Feeding of bone is very useful for the development of skeletal system of growing dogs and also, for the pregnant and nursing bitches. The bones are digested in the stomach by the action of hydrochloric acid secreted by the parietal or oxyntic cells present in the alveoli of the gastric glands. The digestion of bones leaves behind undigested fibrous matrix, which is very useful for the evacuation of bowel. Moreover, feeding of bones in large amount to pet dogs often causes constipation due to large volume of undigested stringy and fibrous residue of bone matrix.

i) Precautions in the feeding of bones

The following points should be kept in mind while offering bones to the pet dogs for chewing :

1. Long bones of fore arm, arm, hind legs or ribs of fresh carcass of lamb, goats or pig should be preferred for the feeding of pet dogs.
2. The amount of bone for feeding should be decided on the basis of age and size of the pet dog.
3. Bones for feeding should be fresh from the healthy animals. Steaming/ partial boiling of bone will be much safe for feeding to avoid the risk of infection.
4. Solid and splintery bones like patella, humerus and femur of large animals and the bones of rabbit, poultry and some of the games should be avoided, as these may cause erosion and laceration of the oral cavity and gut.
5. Feeding of vertebrae of even small animals should be avoided, as these bones sometimes partially choke the oesophagus and cordia of the stomach.
6. Sick dogs particularly that in fever or gastric ailments should not be fed bones.

7.15 Dietary Management of Hepatitis and Jaundice

Feeding of special diet is required for the dogs suffering from hepatitis specially the chronic hepatitis and hepatic cirrhosis. The diets are composed to supply adequate nutrients and energy (ME) for the repair and replacement of liver parenchymal tissue and other associated tissues. The level of dietary protein is kept to meet the maintenance requirement. The excess protein is metabolized to supply energy and the process is taxation on the already damaged liver. The diet should contain high quality protein rich in essential amino acids. The level of protein be preferably at 90-95% of the requirements, and calorie should largely supplied from the highly digestible carbohydrates, e.g. (Table 2).

Table 2.

Diet A:	Braised liver	0.25 lb or g	ME 750 kcal/lb as fed (kcal/ kg)
	Boiled egg, large	60 g	CP 24 %
	Crumbled white bread	3 slice	
	Calcium carbonate	1 teaspoon full	
Diet B:	Boiled rice	2.5 cup or g	ME 690 kcal/lb as fed (kcal/kg)
	Vegetable oil	2 teaspoon full	
	Calcium carbonate	0.25 teaspoon full	
	Potassium chloride	0.25 teaspoon full	
Diet C:	Low fat cottage cheese/paneer	1.5 cup	CP in fed diet 28 g.
	Boiled rice	3.0 cup	
	Cooked liver	1.0 oz	
	Maize oil	1 teaspoon full	
	Dicalcium phosphate	1.0 teaspoon full	
	Vitamin C	250 mg	

For the diets of 18% protein, the quantity of cottage cheese/ paneer is decreased to only 1 cup and boiled rice is increased to 3 cup. Other diets on the basis of chemical composition may be prepared as follows (Table 3):

Table 3.

Diets	Protein	Carbohydrates	Fat	MF (kcal/can/cup)
	16.1/14.8	52.8/61.5	27.3/19.8	612/350
	10.4/9.5	58.4/64.6	27.2/21.0	662/291

Note: ME requirement for maintenance is 132 kcal per kg $W^{0.75.}$ and accordingly

Requirement should be calculated for the different dogs. For other nutrients, see the table on nutrients.

- The diet should not contain rejected meat and fatty tissue.
- Patient should not be forced fed and each meal should be fresh.
- Skimmed milk may be offered.

7.16 Dietary Management of Heart Failure in Dogs

1. Heart failure causes impaired ability to excrete sodium and water loads.
2. Dietary salt restriction is recommended to help fluid accumulation and reduce necessary drug therapy.
3. The degree of sodium restriction depends on the severity of the heart failure.
4. Chloride restriction also considered important.
5. Before signs of heart failure develops, merely avoiding high salt table scraps or treats may be sufficient, although a diet somewhat reduced in sodium is often recommended.
6. Foods that are high in salt include processed meat, liver and kidneys, canned fish, cheese, margarine or butter, canned vegetables, bread, potato chips, pretzels and other munchies, and dogs treat, such as raw hide and biscuits.
7. When clinical heart failure has developed, mild to moderate salt restriction is advised with a sodium intake of about 30 mg/kg/ day (about 0.06% sodium for a canned food or 210-240 mg per

100 g of dry food). Prescription diets for kidney diseases usually provide this recommended level of salt intake.

8. For the advanced heart failure, further sodium restriction can be prescribed in diets (13 mg sodium per kg body weight per day or about 890-1000 mg sodium per 100 g of dry food or 0.025% sodium in the canned foods).
9. The use of drastic sodium restriction (7 mg/kg body weight/ day) exacerbate neurohormonal activation and contribute to hyponetremia in some cases.
10. Most of the commercial dog foods are high in sodium (0.3-1% of sodium on dry matter basis equivalent to over 1100 mg per 100 g dry matter).
11. Foods for the aged (Geriatric) dogs should have lower calorie and protein but some foods still contain a freat deal of salt.
12. Well balanced diets with varying level of sodium restriction are shown in Table 4.
13. A well-balanced diet with adequate calprie and protein is important but inappetence is common in heart failure.
14. Production of cutokines and interleukine 1 B suppress appetite and cause hyper catabolism. Dietary omega 3 fatty acid can reduce the production of these cytokines. The effect of omega 3 fatty acid supplementation in the diets of animals with heart failure are currently being evaluated. These are also useful for the cardiac cachexia.
15. Obesity, on the other hand, increases metabolic demands on the heart and expends blood volume. Increased cardiac filling, stimulation of hypertrophy, increased venous pressure and predisposition to arrythmias may occur. Intrinsic myocardial changes that decrease contractability can also occur with obesity. Mechanical interference with respiration promotes by poventilation. This can contribute to cordiac-pulmonary and complicate pre-existing heart disease. A reducing diet is indicated for grossly overweight pets with heart disease.
16. Supplementation of special nutrients is important in some cases. In some dogs with dilated cardiomyopathy, L-carnitine deficiency has been identified. In some others, taurine

supplementation is also required. Daily administration of 1 to 2g of L-carnitine and 2 to 3 times or 500 mg of taurine two times daily at equal interval has been recommended for the dogs with these deficiencies.

Table 4. Nutrients in different commercial foods

Type of foods	Protein	Fat	Na	Cl	K	Mg	P
Dry foods	17.2	20.9	0.97	0.35	0.72	0.11	0.62
	14.6	19.5	0.21	0.38	0.32	0.06	0.29
	17.7	10.0	0.15	0.52	0.60	0.10	0.51
	16.7	6.9	0.21	0.50	0.60	0.12	0.51
	14.9	16.4	0.34	0.40	0.36	0.08	0.27
	14.4	19.7	0.28	na	0.88	0.09	0.34
	18.6	17.9	0.17	na	1.04	0.10	0.60
Canned food	17.3	28.8	0.10	0.35	0.83	0.15	0.47
	14.8	27.3	0.21	0.25	0.30	0.13	0.11
	17.4	14.0	0.15	0.59	0.63	0.09	0.41
	16.2	12.1	0.26	0.78	0.60	0.08	0.42
	17.8	11.9	0.12	1.27	1.21	0.06	0.40
	16.6	25.3	0.23	0.40	0.33	0.07	0.26
	16.8	21.8	0.24	na	1.50	0.10	0.67
	26.3	38.0	0.10	na	1.50	0.10	0.67
	17.7	21.3	0.11	na	1.31	0.07	0.57

7.17 Dietary Management of Kidney (Renal) related Ailments

Some of the causes of nephritic ailments are hepatitis, initial stages of congestive heart failure, hypertension and encephalitish, besides the composition of diets and source of drinking water. Prolonged inflammatory condition of kidneys and urinary tract often leads to calculi formation causing urolithiasis. The disturbances in elimination of uroliths forming substances ingested in foods is the main cause of renal urolithiasis. Pre-disposing factors of urolithiasis are sudden shifting to dry foods, scanty water intake

Diets for the management of urolithiasis are highly digestible catbohydrated based diets low in protein, calcium, phosphorus, magnesium and sodium. Potassium content should be higher.

7.18 The Aged (Geriatric) Dogs

Following changes are frequently observed with the progressing increase in age and these should be given due consideration in preparation of management schedule of geriatric dogs:

1. Different senses and body weaken.
2. Partial to complete loss of eyesight.
3. Partial to complete loss of hearing.
4. Various degree of muscular weakness.
5. Decrease in indurence (easily fatigued).
6. Becomes incontinent.
7. Dental care may be required.
8. There may be weakening and loss of teeth requiring modification in diets.
9. Treatment of gum may be required.
10. In some dogs, following disorders may occur:
    - i) Nephritis.
    - ii) Heart diseases.
    - iii) Cystitis.
    - iv) Diabetes mellitus, and
    - v) Various types of cancer, etc.
11. Decreased activities.
12. Lowering of the metabolic rate often causes obesity problem.

7.19 Management and Care of Aged (Geriatric) Dog

1. It should be periodically (half yearly or quarterly) examined for the soundness.
2. Health examination should be done by an experienced veterinary doctor, who maimtained the clinical history of dog.
3. Home care is recommended for all but the critically ill and major surgical cases should remain indoor patients.
4. The dog is happier and less worried about itself in home environment.

5. The home routine alongwith gentle and sympathetic care of the owner specially of woman are major care factor.The therapeutic values of tender touch and soft voice of a woman or girl has been well-recognized for early recovery of patients.
6. The diets of patients should be prepared carefully considering the following important factors:
   i) Nutritional requirement.
   ii) Palatability and digestibility.
   iii) Ability of dog to eat and swallow.
   iv) Laxative nature of the food.
   v) The food should be changed gradually, if required.
   vi) Special diets are required in some diseases.
   vii) In some very specific disorder, there may be need of synthetic diets.
7. Fleas has more affinity for the geriatric dogs. Care should be taken for their prevention and elimination in case of infestation.
8. Excess loss of hairs reduces insulation of body and requires protection from cold and chill.
9. Regular grooming will keep the dogs free from ectoparasites and it will also provide opportunity for inspection.

i) Disposal of incurable animals

Affection and attachment of the owner with pets are well-recognized and many times, other family members are overlooked against the pet. But, sometimes pets may suffer from incurable ailments like posterior paralysis in aged German Shepherd and hip dysplasia in some spitz. If a disease is diagnosed incurable and animal suffers from pain and agony, the fate of pet should be decided on humane ground and such animals should be put to painless sleep.Euthenesia is the only solution for providing relief to pet.

□□□

Appendices

Appendix-I. Vaccination schedule

The following vaccination schedule is normally followed, but continuous advances is taking place and accordingly newer vaccines are coming in the market. It is always advised to follow the guidelines of veterinarian for vaccination of pets. Timely vaccination provides protects to pets, owners, neighbours and other animals. Any laxity in vaccination may be disastrous.

Vaccination against (disease)	**Age at vaccination**
Rabies	According to advise of the veterinarian because there are several vaccines with different schedule of vaccination.
Distemper	1st dose before 9 weeks of birth; 2nd at 12 weeks and 3rd or last at 16 weeks of age.
Other diseases	According to instructions on package of vaccine and guidance of the veterinarian.

Appendix-II. Deworming schedule

First deworming: Pregnant bitch is deworme during 6-7 week of gestation.

Second deworming is done at about 2 weeks or as per incidence of worms.

Next deworming should be done only in case of infestation after faecal examination. The drugs used for deworming are harmful substances for healthy animals. These drugs are metabolized in liver and eliminated largely in urine. Thus, both liver and kidneys are taxed.

Appendix-III. Glossary of Dog and Kennel Related Terminology

Dog is considered to be one of the earliest domesticated animal which was developed into different types of large number of breeds through the application of various methods of breeding and selection through several generations for the segregation of desired characteristics. In the process of dog breeding and management, a large number of terminologies for the depicting the characteristics, appearance, behaviour, activities, utility, housing and kennel management have been evolved. It appears that most of these terms are scattered loose and need compilation. Although many of these terms are area specific, indeed their collection may be useful for some institutions. An attempt has been made to collect and compile the available terms in alphabetical sequence.

Achondroplastia	= An abnormal osteogenesis specially the shortening of long bones as in case of Basset hound and Dachshund breeds.
Action	= The act of movement of a dog. This term is used to manage the activities of dog.
Agility	= Quickness.
Agitator	= A person causing irritation or excite the dog.
AKC	= American Kennel Club.
Almond eyes	= The almond-shaped eyes are more common.
Angled	= The bends at joints of hind limbs.
Angulation	= Same as angled.
Apple head	= Domed or convex skull chara.
Apricot	= Somewhat orange coat colour.
Apricot yellow	= Light brownish yellow.
Apricosa	= A frill of different colour on the chest and collar.
Apricot	= Apron
Badger	= Burrowing behaviour. A dog that explore burrow.
Bad mouth	= Abnormal shape of mouth due to faulty dentine.
Balanced diet	= A diet containing all the nutrients in recommended quantity.

Balanced gait	=	Perfect synchronization between the two halves of the body while standing or in action.
Bandy legs	=	Abnormal outwards bending of any one or more legs.
Ban dog	=	A dog kept tied in day light mostly in isolation and let loose in night.
Barking	=	Normal vocalization of any adult dog.
Barrel	=	The size and shape of abdomen.
Barrel chested	=	Excess rounding of rib case.
Barrel hocks	=	Outwards turning of hock joints. Also, called spread backs.
Barren	=	Sterile bitch.
Barrenness	=	Sterility.
Bat ear	=	Ears with broad base, rounded tip and short length with forward turned exposed ear canal.
Bay	=	A howling call generally by a hound in preparation for action.
Beagle	=	Small size hound kept for hunting hares and rabbits.
Beard	=	A tuft of longer hairs than the coat on the chin.
Beauty spot	=	A coloured spot on white blaze on the skull between the ears.
Beeding	=	Tan haircoat on the medial aspect of thigh.
Beefy	=	Heavily muscled hind quarters.
Belton	=	A dense flecking of coloured hairs on white body coat. It appears ticking in short-haired dogs and blurred in long-haired.
Benched	=	Placement of dog on a bench well-secured with chains for inspection at a dog show.
Bird dog	=	Dogs specially trained for hunting birds (mostly in bushes and water source).
BIS	=	Best in show.

Bitch	=	An adult female dog of any age.
Bite	=	1. The act of cutting with teeth. 2. Arrangement of teeth in dogs.
Bites	=	Number of food intake in mouth at a time before chewing and swallowing.
Black	=	Whole colour black coat.
Black penciling on toes	=	Black shading on toes.
Black streak under the jaw	=	
Black and white	=	Body coat of clear black and white patches.
Black, white and red	=	Distinct tricolour (Black, white and red) patches.
Blanket	=	A different solid colour coat over the saddle, generally in hounds.
Blaze	=	A large white patch on the face covering entire or larger area of muzzle from eyes to nose.
Blenheim	=	A toy spaniel with short head and long ears.
Blinker	=	A pointing dog which, upon locating, points the bird.
Blocky	=	Short muzzle appearing drawn in large head in some breds like boxer.
Blooding	=	A practice of allowing young hounds to kill the bait in an effort to increase their hunting desire.
Bloom	=	New crop of glossy coat after shading of old one.
Blue belton	=	Blue flecking on a white coat.
Blue merle	=	Black and grey admixture of hairs as in blue roan.
BOB	=	Best of breed award at a dog show.
Bob tail	=	Birth of tailless puppies or closed docked tail.
Bone/Boned	=	Well-calcified strong and heavier limb bones.

Bonny	=	Strong body frame.
Bossy	=	Muscular full shoulders with raised head and elegant neck.
Brace	=	A pair of dogs, normally of equal size.
Bracelets	=	Ring of hairs left during hair dressing lower part of legs below knee.
Brace mate	=	Member of a brace.
Brach	=	Hunting bitch or hunting breeds.
Breaking	=	Training.
Bred	=	For denoting good typical member of a breed.
Breed	=	A group of fully defined dog as an accepted/ recognized phenotypic traits and behaviour, etc., and capable of producing similar progeny.
Brindle	=	A combination of light and dark colouration of body coat forming irregular stripes. These are usually brown, grey or tan background.
Broken coat	=	Rough and wire haired irregular body coat.
Brood bitch	=	Adult female dog used for breeding.
Brush	=	A bushy fox like tail.
Bull baiting	=	A sport of fight between bull and dog.
Burr	=	Front aspect of inner surface of ear.
Butterfly nose	=	Partially pigmented nose, viz. a black nose with pink area.
Button ear	=	Tightly folded compact ears placed on the skull like a big button and pointing towards the eyes.
Bye or Bye dog	=	Second grade dog.
Canid	=	A member of canine family.
Canines	=	1. A member of canine family.
		2. Long, pointed and pyramidal teeth.
Carlin	=	Old bitch.
Cat feet	=	Short, compact and round feet, as in most of the terrier breeds.

Chap	= Jaws.
Chapping	= Cracking of the surface skin.
Check	= The point at which scent is lost and requiring the help to check,i.e. to find the trail.
Cheeky dog	= Bulging heavy cheeks, as seen in obese dogs.
Cherry nose	= An off colour pink nose. It is a disqualification.
Chestnut	= Reddish brown body coat.
China eyes	= A clear small size blue eyes.
Chiselled face	= A clean and smooth appearance of face down to stop.
Chocolate coat	= Dark brown coat.
Choke chain	= A special chain with gliding collar arranged to loose or tight as per Control of the handler's grip.
Chop	= Special voice of some short, sharp bearing notes of a trailing hand.
Chopped	= When a fox is killed by the dog before breaking cover.
Chops	= Jowl or pendulous flesh of lips.
Clip	= Hair dressing.
Clipping	= Knuckling or hiting of posterior aspect of fore legs with hind legs during motion.
Cloddy	= Low set broad or round and heavy dogs.
Close coupled	= Comparatively short from wethers to hip bone or upto set on the tail.
Coarse dog	= An untrained and unruly dog.
Coarse hair	= Rough, thick and hard hairs of body coat. Generally outer coat of double coated dogs.
Coat	= Hair cover of the body.
Coat colour	= The colour of hairs covering the body.
Coat foot	= Short, compact and rounded foot with close set and well-arched toes.

Cobby	=	Muscular compact body with short back, deep chest and well-sprung ribs.
Collar	=	A white marking around the neck on coloured body coat.
Condition	=	General appearance of the dog.
Corded/Cords	=	Hairs curled around central core of hairs forming many hanging cords. It is different from mats.
Couples	=	A pair of hounds of same breed.
Coupling	=	The length of ventral aspect of body between last rib and anterior of symphysis pubis.
Covering ground	=	The strides involving fore legs and hind legs.
Cow hocked	=	A deformity of hind legs showing inwards bending of hock joints and outwards deflection of feet.
Crabbing	=	Side way movements made by standing dog.
Crank tail	=	A hanging tail.
Crest	=	Dorsal line of neck extending from shoulders to base of occiput.
Crop	=	Hunter's whip.
Cropping	=	Cutting of ear leathers for providing erect shape. It is not accepted in many countries and many states or communes in many countries.
Crossbred	=	Offsprings of sire and dam of different breeds.
Croup	=	Area between posterior end of lion and base of the tail.
Crown	=	The top of the skull between the ear base, i.e. occiput.
Crying	=	Noise made due to pain.
Cryptorchid	=	A male in which one or both testicles are not desended in the scrotum.
Cullote	=	Very long hairs on the posterior aspect of thighs.

Cur	= An undefined or mongrel dog.
Cushion	= Thickness of the upper lip in Pekingese, Boxer and few other breeds.
Dam	= Mother.
Dappled	= Mottled markings of different colours without any predominating colour.
Dead grass	= A dull straw colour dog.
Deciduous teeth	= Milk teeth.
Dental	= Of teeth.
Dental formula	= Depiction of arrangement of total teeth.
Dentition	= Eruption of teeth.
Dew claw	= Additional toes on the pasterns.
Dewlap	= Loose skin on ventral aspect of neck, which may extend upto brisket.
Dexterity	= Cleverness.
Dish face	= A shallow concave forehead extending down to nasal bone.
Dock	= Amputed tail stump.
Docking	= Specialized amputation of tail. May be cosmetic or clinical.
Dog	= A member of dog family irrespective of age, sex and definition.
Dolichocephalic	= Long headed dog.
Double coat	= Two different types of coats on the body. Under coat is wool fibre and outer coat is made of long and coarse hairs in breeds of cold zone.
Down faced	= Downward curving of nasal bone from top to tip of the nose.
Down pasterns	= Bending of fore legs due to weakness or deformity of metacarpus.
Drag	= A trail made by drawing a bag of animal scent (generally faeces). It is used for training hounds for fast race and search.

Drag hounds	=	Hounds hunting a scented trail.
Draft or Draught dog	=	Working dog.
Dressing	=	Preparation of dogs including hair clipping for improvement in look.
Drop ears	=	Hanging ears; may be pendulous also.
Dropping	=	Prefix used for hanging ears or tail.
Droppings	=	Faeces.
Dropped muscle	=	Rupture of an inner loin or shoulder muscle.
Dropper	=	A crossbred bird dog.
Dry neck	=	Taut skin.
Dual champian	=	Champion in two different events at same show.
Duddley (Dudley) nose	=	Light brown or flesh colour nose.
Dysplasia	=	Loose set hip joint; mostly a congenital anamoly.
Ear carriage	=	Device for correction of folded ear in a breed of characteristic prick ear.
Ears	=	External ears or pinnae or leathers. Leathers is used for long hanging ears.
Earth	=	The burrow of fox.
Eclampsia	=	Nursing bitch.
Ectopion	=	Outwards directed eyes.
Entropion	=	Inwards directed eyes.
Even bite	=	Upper and lower row of teeth oppose.
Ewe neck	=	Concave neck.
Eye teeth	=	Upper canine teeth.
Faking	=	Manipulation of appearance for hiding defects or projecting an artificially made desired trait.
Fall	=	Long hairs falling on the face.
Fangs	=	Canine teeth.

Fantum pregnancy	= Pseudopregnancy or false pregnancy.
Farinaceous foods	= Starchy foods containing flour.
Feathering	= Long hairs or tuft of long hairs on body. Specially on legs, tain and thighs.
Felted coat	= Mat forming (not cord forming) of coat.
Fetch	= Caution for retrieving or act of retrieving.
Fiddle	= The feet turned inwards and elbows turned outwards.
Flag or flag tail	= Feathering of under surface of tail with longer hairs towards the root and gradually decreasing length towards the tip.
Flank	= An area on body surrounded by lumbar spines, last rib and anterior of hip bone.
Flare	= A blaze wider at the top of the skull than between the eyes.
Flat sided	= Narrow chest due to less sprung ribs.
Flecked	= Shading of the coat when lightly ticked with other colours.
Flew	= Pendulous upper jaw overlapping the lower lip to various degree.
Flush	= Driving away prey (birds or animals) from cover.
Flying ears	= Folded or semi prick ears, when stand erect form.
	= Resting place of hares and rabbits.
Form	= Resting place of hare.
Foster mother	= Nursing bitch other than the mother.
Foul colour	= A typical coat colour or markings.
French front	= Fiddle front.
Frill	= Long feathering around the neck with shorter hairs at the throat.

Fringe	=	Feathering.
Frog face	=	An overshot upper jaw and extended nose.
Front	=	Anterior visible part of the body.
Full cry	=	Noise made by whole pack, when chasing the quarry.
Furnishing	=	Profuse long hairs on certain part of the body specially the fore face.
Furrow	=	A line running from center of the occiput to stop on the fore head.
Futurity	=	An event for young dogs which have been nominated pre-natal or at birth.
Gait	=	Natural style of standing and movement.
Gay	=	Tail carried curled over the back.
Gestation	=	Pregnancy.
Giving tongue	=	Hounds when got onto a scent of prey.
Gnawing	=	Chewing a hard object, viz. bone or emitted bone.
Goose rump	=	Steep or sloping rump.
Grizzle	=	Bluish grey colour.
Grooming	=	Cleaning of body.
Guard dogs	=	Dogs specialized for protection.
Guard hairs	=	Long hairs or outer coat for concealing the under coat.
Gun barrel front	=	Straight fore legs.
Gun dog	=	Hunting dogs.
Gun shy	=	Dog becoming nervous after seeing a gun or hearing a gun shot.
Hackles	=	Erected state of hairs on neck and back in a threatened dog due to fright or uncertainity.
Hard dog	=	Terriers which are determined fighters and diggers.

Hard mouthed = A hunting dog which fears the retrieved game.

Hare foot = Feet with longer and well apart toes.

Hare lip = Cleft upper lip or palate.

Harlequin = Patched or pied colouration of a white or black ground colour like the dress of bafoons.

Harness = Appliances used for controlling the dogs and of working dogs.

Harrier = A small fox hound kept for hunting the hare.

Harsh coat = A stiff coat of straight or wire hairs.

Haw = Nictitating membrane.

Heat = Oestrum.

Height = The measurement from ground to top of the withers.

Hermaphrodite = Presence of complete or incomplete organs of both sexes in the same animal.

Hocks = Joint formed of femer and tibia bones.

Hog mouth = Under shot upper jaw.

Hounds = Dogs capable to pursue the game, prevent escape and finally kill.

Hound markings = White, tan or black patches on the body, as in many hounds.

Huckle bones = Top of the hip bones.

Hunting = To catch prey or game.

Hunting crop = A whip carried by hunters during hunting operations.

Hup = Command given to a Spaniel to halt and sit.

Husky = Term for mongrel in Arctic America.

In breeding = Mating among very close relatives within the family.

ICD = Indian classification of dogs.

Incisors = Front teeth on jaws before canines.

In season	= A bitch in oestrous or heat.
Isabella	= Fawn or greyish yellow colour.
Jaws	= The bones of face bearing the teeth.
Jowl	= Fleshy loose part of the ventral aspect of lower jaw.
Kampf	= It is a method of ear cropping living behind only cartilaginous part.
KCI	= Kennel club of India.
Kink tail	= A short twist or bend in the tail.
Kiss marks	= Tan spots on cheeks and eyebrows.
Lemon colour	= Light yellow colour with greenish tinge.
Lay back	= The angle at which the shoulder blade departs from perpendicular.
Lean head	= A head with little flesh and tight skin.
Leash	= A thong or line for holding dog.
Leathers	= Long drooping ear flaps.
Leonite	= Lion like.
Level bite	= Edge to edge meeting of teeth (Pincer bite).
Liam	= Lead or leash.
Lights	= Lungs with trachea and bronchial tubes.
Limb	= Entire leg from top to toes.
Line breeding	= Mating between close relatives of a family in sequence.
Lippy	= Total number of pups in a litter.
Litter	= Total puppies of one whelping.
Litters	= Waste materials of kennel.
Loaded shoulders	= Abnormally heavy shoulders.
Lock up or tie	= Tail to tail joining of dog and bitch at third stage of mating.

Loins	= An area of body from last rib to anterior of the pelvic.
Lumbar	= An area between last thoracic and first sacral vertebra.
Lurcher	= A crossbred hound.
Magyar	= Hungarian.
Maiden	= An unmated or open female dog.
Manteltiger	= Black forms of mantle with pure white neck, legs and tip of the tail.
Mantle	= Dark shaded portion of hairs on the back and sides like blanket.
Marbled	= Mottled couleration of coat.
Mask	= A different color of face than the coat colour.
Match	= Informal dog show.
Melena	= Dark tarry faeces indicating haemorrhage in anterior part of the gut.
Merle	= Blue and grey colour mixed hairs of coat with black streaks.
Milk teeth	= Deciduous teeth.
Miscelleneous class	= Dogs not falling in the recommended classes of kennel.
Mis marked	= Deviation of coat colour from the standard.
Molar teeth	= Cheek teeth.
Molera/Mollera	= Deformed ossification of skull.
Mongrel	= Non-descript dog.
Moulting	= Normal shading of coat.
Music	= The vocalization of hounds in full cry.
Mute	= A silently running hound on the trail.
Muzzle	= Lower part of face down the stop.
Nick	= Transmission of desired phenotypic traits from parents to off spring.

Non-slip retriever	= A dog that stays at heel, marks the fall of game and retrives to command.
Nose	= Olfactory organ.
(To) Nose	= Ability of a dog in scenting and called as: (i) great nose = very sharp, (ii) poor nose = low ability and (iii) no nose = failed ability.
Obese	= Fatty dog.
Obesity	= Excessive fattyness.
Occiput	= The upper most part of skull.
Orbit	= Bony cavity in skull for eyes.
Out cross	= Mating between unrelated mates of same breed.
Out of elbow	= Elbows turning out of the body.
Otter tail	= A tail thick at the root with hairs parted on the under side but not flagged.
Over hang	= Prominent eyebrow looming over a pushed in face.
Pace	= Movement of legs of one side.
Pack	= A group of hound or hunting dogs.
Pad	= (i) Sole of the dog; and (ii) The Fox's foot.
Paddling	= Moving too wide in front with feet mostly turning out, as they are lifted at the end of the step.
Paper foot	= Thin soled flat foot.
Parent club	= National breed club.
Parrot mouth	= Overshot mouth.
Parti-coloured	= Patches of two or more colours.
Pasterns	= Metacarpus in fore legs and metatarsus in hind legs.
Patches	= Large size solid colour spot(s) on body coat.
Patella	= Knee cap, a blunt triangular solid bone.
Peak	= Occiput.

Pedigree	=	Written record of parentage. Should be at least upto Great grand parents.
Penciling	=	Blue line on tan colour toes.
Pied or piebald	=	Parti-coloured.
Pigeon breast	=	A chest with a short protruding breast bone.
Pigeon toed	=	Inwards turned toes.
Pig eye	=	Abnormally small eyes.
Pig jaw	=	Grossly undershot upper jaw.
Pig mouth	=	Undershot upper jaw.
Piggish	=	Obese dog.
Pigmentation	=	Colouration of skin, hairs and other body parts.
Pile	=	Dense under coat.
Pincer bite	=	Level bite.
Pinscher	=	Terrier in German language.
Plating	=	Placing one foot in front of another with a twisting motion.
Plumb	=	Perfectly vertical fore legs.
Plumes	=	Soft and long hairs on tail, as in brush tail.
Point	=	Rigid posture adopted by a hunting dog to reveal the location of game.
Points	=	Colour of hairs on the legs, face, ears and tail.
Poke	=	To carry neck at an abnormal low angle.
Pompon	=	Circular tuft of hairs at the end of tail.
Pregnancy	=	Gestation.
Pre-molar	=	Cheek teeth between canines and molars.
Pre-potency	=	Resemblence of off springs with the parent.
Prick ears	=	Erect ears.
Pseudopregnancy	=	It is false pregnancy showing signs of pregnancy. Synonym is Fantum pregnancy.

Pug	=	Flattened muzzle dog.
Puli	=	A Hungarian breed of dog.
Pumi	=	Same as Puli.
Pup/Puppy	=	Young dogs.
Puppy coat	=	The first body coat.
Puppying	=	Whelping.
Pup sac	=	Foetal membrane covering each pup of litter.
Quality	=	Conformation and appearance of dogs.
Quick	=	The dead nail portion in dogs.
Racy dog	=	Tall dog of light built.
Rag tail	=	A tail with hairless tail.
Rangy dog	=	A tall, long and slender dog.
Ranula	=	A swelling under the tongue.
Rat tail	=	A tail with thick base covered with curls and bare tip.
Red roan	=	Uniform admixture of red and white hairs of body coat.
Ribbed up	=	Deep chest or well sprung ribs.
Ring	=	An area demarked for judging the dogs at show.
Ring stern	=	Curled tail as ring tail.
Ring tail	=	Curled tail carried over the back.
Roach back	=	Convex arched back.
Roan	=	Uniform mixture of coloured hairs with white hairs.
Roman nose	=	Convex and long nose bridge.
Rose ear	=	A twisted or folded ear exposing the inner surface.
Rounding	=	Cutting of ear leather to make rounded shape.
Rudder	=	Whip like tail as in Grey hound and Rampur hound.

Ruff	= Frill, i.e. thick and long hairs around the neck.
Running mute	= A hound hunting without giving tongue.
Sable	= A bright black hair lacing on lighter coat.
Sabre tail	= Almost half curled tail.
Saddle back	= Excessively long back.
Saddle mark	= A black or solid colour marking on the back resembling a saddle but smaller than the blanket.
Sapling	= An untested Grey hound pup (10-18 months old).
Scent	= Hounds hunt their quarry by scent. It is never called smell.
Scissors bite	= Outer surface of lower incisors are covered by inner surface of upper incisors, when mouth is close or biting.
Screw tail	= A short and screw form twisted tail.
Sedge	= Dead grass coat colour.
Self colour	= A single whole colour except shading.
Self markings	= A single colour coat with white or pale markings on the chest, feet and either tip or under surface of tail.
Semi-prick	= Erect ears with bend tips.
Service	= Mating in a stud under supervision.
Services	= Pet shop.
Set up	= Display of dog in a show ring.
Sex play	= An oversexual dog (A nuisance & embarrassing behaviour of a pet dog).
Shedding	= Moulting.
Shelly	= A shallow and narrow body with too much tuck up and generally an insufficient amount of bones.
Sickle hocks	= Well let down hocks with strong angulation of both stifles and hocks.

Sickle tail	= A shallow curved tail with upward tip.
Simmering	= In a restrained state.
Single colour	= Whole colour.
Single tracking	= Dog moving his feet close together to achieve perfect balance specially during trot.
Skirting	= A trailing dog which runs along its brace mate not trying to pick up scent until the turn.
Slab sided	= A dog with narrow chest due to less sprung ribs.
Smooth coat	= Coat of uniform short and dense hairs.
Snarling	= Confused.
Snipy	= Weak, thin and pointed muzzle.
Soft mouth	= A dog which retrieves without injuring the prey or farm animal by biting and tearing the subjects.
Soundness	= Status of health.
Spayed	= Surgically sterilized bitch.
Spaying	= Surgery for sterilization of bitch.
Spactacles	= A dark marking or shading around the eyes like spectacles.
Spitz	= A square shaped dog.
Splashed	= Patches of white colour on solid coat or vice versa.
Splay foot	= Flat foot with spread toes and paper pad.
Spread	= Arched fore legs as in Bulldog.
Squirrel tail	= A tail carried upright and then falling flat on the back.
Standard dog	= Specimen true to breed standard as per kennel rules.
Stand off coat	= Long coat standing out from the body, as in Apso breed.
Staring coat	= Bad or poor coat.
Stern	= Whip like tail of a sporting or hunting breed.

Stifle	= A joint formed of distal end of femur and proximal end of tibia bones.
Stilted	= Gait of a straight hoch dog.
Sting tail	= A tail tapering to a fine point.
Stop	= A depression at the junction of skull and nasal bones at the level of eyes.
Stopping earth	= Filling in earths for stopping a fox to enter its burrow.
Straight hocked	= Insufficiently angled hock joint.
Stripping	= Pulling out excess and unwanted hairs for thinning and coat smoothness.
Stud dog	= Entire standard male kept for breeding.
Superciliary arches	= Frontal bones of the skull forming the eyebrows.
Sway back	= Concave curvature of the back from withers to croup.
Swill	= Food wastes containing meat scraps.
Symmetry	= Growth of dogs as per standards for breeds.
Tail	= The organ made of coccigeal vertebrae.
Tailing	= Docking.
Terrier	= Dogs with habit of digging, pursuing and driving game out of burrow.
Tassels	= Corded hairs of dog.
Team	= A group of more than two working dogs.
Terrier front	= Straight profile of the front.
Texture	= Quality of coat hairs.
Thong	= A strip of leather used for restraining dogs.
Throaty or throatiness	= Loose hanging jowl.
Through back	= Unexpected similarity of puppy with a distant relative.

Thumb marks	=	Black marks on pastern.
Ticked	=	Small and distinct black or colourered marks on a white ground coat.
Timber bone	=	Leg bone.
To given gue	=	Call of hound on trail.
Top knot	=	A tuft of long hairs on the top of head in some breeds.
Top line	=	Dorsal line from withers to root of the tail.
Toy dog	=	Tiny breeds of dog.
Trace	=	Dark stripe along the back characteristic for pug.
Trail	=	To hunt by following ground scent or by scent emitted.
Triangular ears	=	Ears with broad base and pointed tip.
Tri-colour	=	Three colour body coat.
Trim	=	Clipping and plucking of irregular and unwanted hairs.
Trout marks	=	Small reddish markings on the light colour coat.
Trumpet	=	Dog's temple or the hollow on either side of the skull.
Tuck up	=	Pulled loin or lack of depth of loin.
Tulip ear	=	Slightly forward curved ears.
Tufter	=	Two or three couples of the oldest and wisest stag hounds sent into cover to search and drive out the deer.
Type	=	As per official standard of a kennel.
Under coat	=	Fine hair woolly soft body coat beneath the coarse outer coat in double coated dogs.
Under shot	=	Upper jaw shorter than the lower jaw. Also, called hog mouth.
Varminty	=	A keen and piercing expression like a fox.
Vent	=	Anal opening.

Viciousness	=	The vice of biting.
Wall eye	=	Complete or part of iris of one or both eye balls either white or pale.
Weaving	=	Crossing the fore feet or hind feet during motion.
Wheaten	=	Fawn or pale yellow body coat tending towards red.
Wheel back	=	Strongly arched back.
Whelping	=	Parturition or delivery.
Whip tail	=	Tail carried stiffly at the level of back or doral line.
Whiskers	=	The neat and tidy beard of terriers, which is much less dense than the full beard.
Wire haired	=	Rough and twisted hairs.
Withers	=	The dorsal border of shoulder.
Worrying	=	Attacking or chasing.
Wrench	=	To bend the hare from its line at less than right angle while chasing.
Wrinkles	=	Loose skin folds on the face or any part of body.
Yelp	=	To give a quick, sharp and shrilled cry.
Zygoma	=	Grinding and teeth baring action of dog.

❏❏❏

Twice as nice: Barbra Streisand cloned beloved dog

AFP

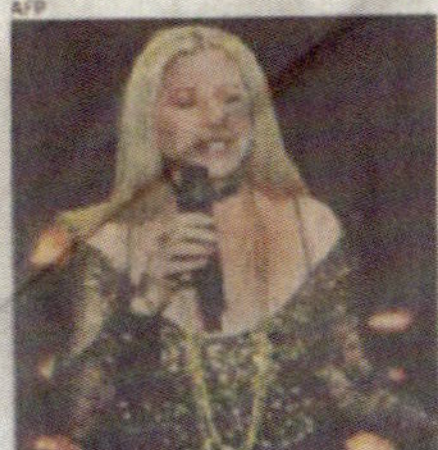

Streisand's Coton de Tulear dog Samantha died in 2017

Los Angeles: "If we had the chance to do it all again, tell me would we, could we?" Barbra Streisand had a hit singing this question in 'The Way We Were', but when it comes to getting a new pet she does not have to wonder.

The 'Funny Girl' singer and actress had her beloved 14-year-old Coton de Tulear dog Samantha cloned after her death in 2017, and now has two new pups. Coton de Tulear is a small breed and has a cotton-like coat.

Streisand told Hollywood trade publication 'Variety' in an interview published on Tuesday that cells were taken from the mouth and stomach of Samantha.

"They have different personalities," Streisand said, adding, "I'm waiting for them to get older so I can see if they have her brown eyes and her seriousness."

Streisand said when the cloned dogs arrived, she dressed them in red and lavender to tell them apart, which is how they got their names — Miss Scarlett and Miss Violet.

The Oscar and Tony winning actress, 75, said while waiting for their arrival, she became smitten with another dog who was a distant relation of Samantha.

If the possibility of cloning your dog intrigues you, there is good news: You do not have to be a famous actor, director, producer and writer to have it done.

South Korean researchers announced that they had cloned a dog for the first time in 2005, after almost three years of work and more than 1,000 eggs. With help from a yellow Labrador retriever who served as the surrogate mother, a cloned male Afghan hound named Snuppy was born. (Snuppy, of course, stood for "Seoul National University puppy.")

By 2008, a California company had partnered with a South Korean laboratory and made plans to auction off chances to clone five dogs. Later that year, 'The New York Times' reported that the first three puppies from the group had been born in South Korea. Two 2015 reports from 'Business Insider' and 'NPR' detail the work of Sooam Biotech, a lab in South Korea, which had cloned more than 600 dogs. NYT & AGENCIES

Source: The Times of India, New Delhi, Thursday, March 1, 2018

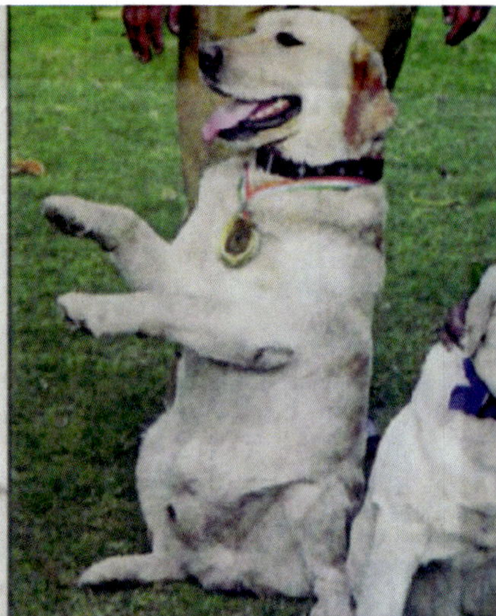

BOW WOWS: The canine force of Delhi Police made its mark at the recently concluded all India Police Duty meet in Chennai. Apart from winning an Asadharan Karya Puraskar, the team also won gold in the tracking event and bronze medals in explosive-detection and videography categories. The dog squad won gold in tracking event for the first time, with its dog 'Babu' and handler, constable Pawan Kumar Yadav, bagging the medal in their first participation

Source: The Times of India, New Delhi, Friday, March 16, 2018

Dog on duty for metro Security

'Girl' canines on the job to secure metro

Sidhartha.Roy
@timesgroup.com

New Delhi: Maya, Ruby, Stella, Nikki, Alice and Heena are part of an elite all-female squad of CISF. Most of these highly trained "girls" are just about a year old. What makes them unique? They are the latest addition to CISF's metro canine squad.

CISF's dog squad is now 60 strong with eight new recruits. It's the need of the hour as the network is expanding, and there may be more additions with further expansion. Pure-bred puppies are bought and sent to BSF Academy in Tekanpur, Madhya Pradesh. They are trained to obey commands, sniff out explosives and contraband, and adapt to the crowded environment of metro trains and stations.

Labradors and German shepherds are the most preferred breeds. A Labrador pup can cost up to Rs 25,000. Cocker spaniels and golden retrievers come next in the preference ladder. There are 31 Labradors in the squad, 17 German shepherds, 10 cocker spaniels and two golden retrievers.

Trained dogs are sent back to CISF and their handlers chosen. "Volunteers are primarily those who love dogs," said a CISF officer. The handlers also name the dogs, which get no salary or rank but get food, care and shelter.

There's a reason why only female dogs are in the squad. "Male dogs can be more aggressive and we can't allow that in a metro environment. More importantly, male dogs often get distracted while on the job, particularly when they are in heat," the officer said.

The dogs are kept in kennels at different facilities near the metro corridors. Their day starts early with grooming and physical training. Each dog does a four-hour shift, and 20 dogs are always present in the metro network at most times. Some dogs are also kept on standby at night for emergencies. When a dog sniffs an explosive, it sits tight at the spot.

But as the metro surface is slippery, dogs find it difficult to get a grip while walking resulting in some cases their legs getting bent, the officer said.

Each dog has a career span of 10 years, after which it retires and is donated to an NGO. Many dogs are bought for security work in malls.

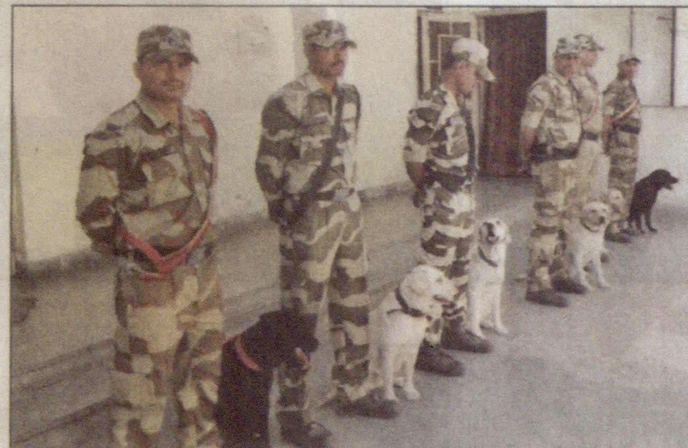

SQUAD ON DUTY: Each dog does a four-hour shift, and 20 dogs are always present in the metro network at most times

Source: Sunday Times of India, New Delhi, March 18, 2018

There's a glass ceiling in canine world too

Reuters

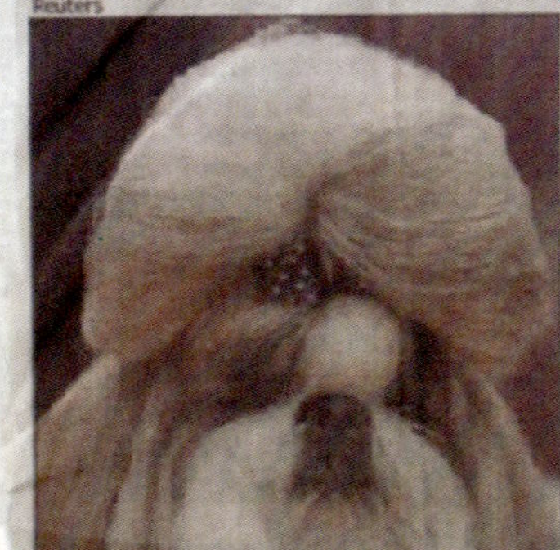

A Shih Tzu at a media preview event for the Westminster Kennel Club Dog Show in NYC

After the German shepherd Rumor won the top prize at last year's Westminster Kennel Club Dog Show in New York, she had her first litter of puppies and retired, like many female show dogs.

By contrast, most top male show dogs can keep competing for years, and it is no coincidence that they also win 'Best in Show' in the annual competition far more often than females, breeders and handlers said as they prepared for this year's show, which opens on Monday in New York.

"Now she won't show again, she's done," said Gail Miller Bisher, a spokeswoman for the Westminster Kennel Club, referring to Rumor. "But males can keep going. They can... continue showing and keep their coat and keep their shape of body and all that."

Female dogs have snared 'Best in Show' at Westminster 39 times since the award was first given in 1907. On the other hand, males have been victorious 71 times.

A dog's peak age for competition is three to five years old, which also happens to be prime breeding age for females, said Kimberly Calvacca, a professional handler and breeder from New York. Females are less likely to compete at Westminster.

This year, there were 1,220 female competitors and 1,699 male challengers enrolled in most categories, including vying to be named top dog on Tuesday. A female competitor's "heat" cycle brings changes in temperament and hormones that can also hurt her chances of winning the show. Depending on the breed, a female dog in season will shed her coat, leaving a female dog less impressive looking than male peers. Those kinds of changes can knock her out of the competition for months.

Betty-Anne Stenmark, the sole judge of this year's 'Best in Show' competition at Westminster, said appearance was important when it comes to picking a world champion. But she denied the cards are stacked in favour of males. REUTERS

Source: The Times of India, New Delhi, Saturday, February 10, 2018

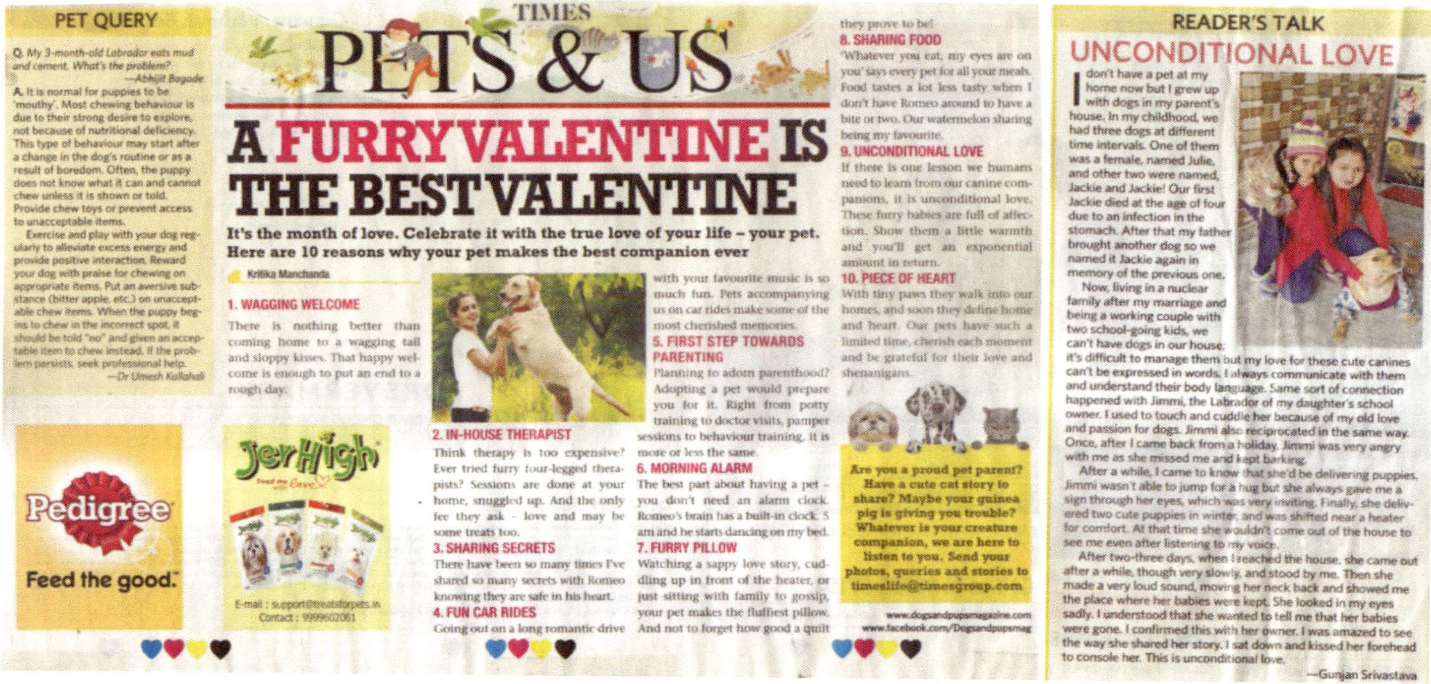

PET QUERY

Q. My 3-month-old Labrador eats mud and cement. What's the problem?
—Abhijit Bagade

A. It is normal for puppies to be 'mouthy'. Most chewing behaviour is due to their strong desire to explore, not because of nutritional deficiency. This type of behaviour may start after a change in the dog's routine or as a result of boredom. Often, the puppy does not know what it can and cannot chew unless it is shown or told. Provide chew toys or prevent access to unacceptable items.

Exercise and play with your dog regularly to alleviate excess energy and provide positive interaction. Reward your dog with praise for chewing on appropriate items. Put an aversive substance (bitter apple, etc.) on unacceptable chew items. When the puppy begins to chew in the incorrect spot, it should be told "no" and given an acceptable item to chew instead. If the problem persists, seek professional help.
—Dr Umesh Kallahali

TIMES PETS & US

A FURRY VALENTINE IS THE BEST VALENTINE

It's the month of love. Celebrate it with the true love of your life – your pet. Here are 10 reasons why your pet makes the best companion ever

Kritika Manchanda

1. WAGGING WELCOME

There is nothing better than coming home to a wagging tail and sloppy kisses. That happy welcome is enough to put an end to a rough day.

2. IN-HOUSE THERAPIST

Think therapy is too expensive? Ever tried furry four-legged therapists? Sessions are done at your home, snuggled up. And the only fee they ask - love and may be some treats too.

3. SHARING SECRETS

There have been so many times I've shared so many secrets with Romeo knowing they are safe in his heart.

4. FUN CAR RIDES

Going out on a long romantic drive with your favourite music is so much fun. Pets accompanying us on car rides make some of the most cherished memories.

5. FIRST STEP TOWARDS PARENTING

Planning to adorn parenthood? Adopting a pet would prepare you for it. Right from potty training to doctor visits, pamper sessions to behaviour training, it is more or less the same.

6. MORNING ALARM

The best part about having a pet – you don't need an alarm clock. Romeo's brain has a built-in clock. 5 am and he starts dancing on my bed.

7. FURRY PILLOW

Watching a sappy love story, cuddling up in front of the heater, or just sitting with family to gossip, your pet makes the fluffiest pillow. And not to forget how good a quilt they prove to be!

8. SHARING FOOD

'Whatever you eat, my eyes are on you' says every pet for all your meals. Food tastes a lot less tasty when I don't have Romeo around to have a bite or two. Our watermelon sharing being my favourite.

9. UNCONDITIONAL LOVE

If there is one lesson we humans need to learn from our canine companions, it is unconditional love. These furry babies are full of affection. Show them a little warmth and you'll get an exponential amount in return.

10. PIECE OF HEART

With tiny paws they walk into our homes, and soon they define home and heart. Our pets have such a limited time, cherish each moment and be grateful for their love and shenanigans.

Are you a proud pet parent? Have a cute cat story to share? Maybe your guinea pig is giving you trouble? Whatever is your creature companion, we are here to listen to you. Send your photos, queries and stories to timeslife@timesgroup.com

www.dogsandpupsmagazine.com
www.facebook.com/Dogsandpupsmag

READER'S TALK

UNCONDITIONAL LOVE

I don't have a pet at my home now but I grew up with dogs in my parent's house. In my childhood, we had three dogs at different time intervals. One of them was a female, named Julie, and other two were named, Jackie and Jackie! Our first Jackie died at the age of four due to an infection in the stomach. After that my father brought another dog so we named it Jackie again in memory of the previous one.

Now, living in a nuclear family after my marriage and being a working couple with two school-going kids, we can't have dogs in our house; it's difficult to manage them but my love for these cute canines can't be expressed in words. I always communicate with them and understand their body language. Same sort of connection happened with Jimmi, the Labrador of my daughter's school owner. I used to touch and cuddle her because of my old love and passion for dogs. Jimmi also reciprocated in the same way. Once, after I came back from a holiday, Jimmi was very angry with me as she missed me and kept barking.

After a while, I came to know that she'd be delivering puppies. Jimmi wasn't able to jump for a hug but she always gave me a sign through her eyes, which was very inviting. Finally, she delivered two cute puppies in winter, and was shifted near a heater for comfort. At that time she wouldn't come out of the house to see me even after listening to my voice.

After two-three days, when I reached the house, she came out after a while, though very slowly, and stood by me. Then she made a very loud sound, moving her neck back and showed me the place where her babies were kept. She looked in my eyes sadly. I understood that she wanted to tell me that her babies were gone. I confirmed this with her owner. I was amazed to see the way she shared her story. I sat down and kissed her forehead to console her. This is unconditional love.

—Gunjan Srivastava

Source: Sunday Times of India, New Delhi, February 11, 2018

□□□